Screening in Child Health Care

Report of the Dutch Working Party
on Child Health Care

Micha de Winter
Mariëlle Balledux
José de Mare
Ruud Burgmeijer

Radcliffe Medical Press
Oxford • New York

© 1995 Micha de Winter, Mariëlle Balledux, José de Mare, Ruud Burgmeijer

Radcliffe Medical Press Ltd
18 Marcham Road, Abingdon, Oxon OX14 1AA, UK

Radcliffe Medical Press, Inc.
141 Fifth Avenue, New York, NY 10010, USA

British Library Cataloguing in Publication Data

A catalogue record for this book is available from the British Library.

ISBN 1 857751 50 7

Library of Congress Cataloging-in-Publication Data is available.

Translated by BSA Texts, © March 1994
Typeset by Marksbury Typesetting Ltd, Midsomer Norton, Bath, UK
Printed and bound by Biddles Ltd., Guildford and King's Lynn

Contents

Introduction
a critical evaluation of Dutch preventive Child Health Care

Child Health Care for the pre-school age range has in many Western countries increasingly grown into a subject of scientific, social and political debate over the last few years. In Britain, the Joint Working Party on Child Health Surveillance published a report in 1989, in which existing services were critically examined and recommendations were made for future practice (Hall et al. 1989). In the Netherlands as well, there were strong reasons to do this. To put it briefly: Dutch Child Health Care, which for a long time had enjoyed wide social support and appreciation, found itself faced with the obligation to legitimize itself under the influence of new political developments; society demanded a more accurate insight into the results of its efforts. Within this context, the project called 'Integral Evaluation of Child Health Care' was initiated. The Board of the National Association for Community Nursing and Home Care[1] commissioned the Centre for Research and Development of Youth Health Care and Youth Social Work of the University of Utrecht to subject the Dutch Child Health Care system to a scientific study. In this study special attention had to be paid to quality, cost effectiveness and general effectiveness, efficiency, and shortcomings in care. The project was financially supported by the Ministry of Welfare, Public Health and Cultural Affairs, and the Foundation for Research and Development of Social Services. Even before the project was wound up in the middle of 1992, another political discussion flared up, shaking the sector to its foundations: at the end of 1991 Christian Democrat and Labour MPs proposed a motion to transfer the responsibility for the Child Health Care system, plus its financing, to local authorities. The Integral Evaluation Project then took on a somewhat different aspect. While it was initially meant to provide a better insight into the effects of the health care system, its results were now expected to play

---

[1]For a long time 'Cross Associations' (Kruisverenigingen) have been active in the Netherlands in the fields of social and preventive medicine and home nursing on behalf of their members as well as of the general public. The National Cross Association (Nationale Kruisvereniging) represented the regional cross associations at national level. In 1990 the National Cross Association merged with the National Council for Home Help (Centrale Raad voor de Gezinsverzorging) to form the National Association for community Nursing and Home Care (Landelijke Vereniging voor Thuiszorg), established at Bunnik. In this book the regional organizations will be referred to as 'Community Health Care'.

an important part in the political decision-making process on the question of whether the Child Health Care system remains a nationwide, guaranteed basic facility or becomes subject to locally established priorities.

The objective of the project was formulated as follows:
'On the basis of existing national and international research material, the project aims to arrive at a scientifically sound assessment of the present Child Health Care system, on which proposals for changes in care, if necessary and if possible, can be based. Should the study show, on the basis of national and international data, that a scientifically sound assessment cannot be made because parts of the research material are insufficient, then recommendations for further research, such as cost-effectiveness studies, will need to be formulated. In such a case this investigation must be considered a preliminary study, which on the one hand ought to yield material to reach a scientific consensus on the Child Health Care system, and on the other hand must be viewed as a study that will enable the programming and attuning of further research into the desirable content and organization of the Child Health Care system. This integral study of Dutch Child Health Care (in its relation to child health surveillance programmes in other countries) should yield conclusions and recommendations relating to:

- the necessary and desirable content of the Dutch Child Health Care system, if possible on the basis of cost-effectiveness data

- the frequency with which various studies are to be carried out

- the necessary expertise

- all-round or specialist district health care within the Child Health Care system

- the procedures of quality control and quality improvement

- possibilities for greater parental involvement in Child Health Care.

In view of the breadth and complexity of the above-mentioned issues, the project was centred around an 'expert committee', an independent expert working party, which was composed on the basis of scientific, professional and/or social authority in the area of youth health care or related areas. Besides the professional groups directly involved, experts from relevant medical and social science disciplines, the government, chief medical inspectors, advisory bodies, medical insurance companies, Community Health Care organizations, municipal and regional health services, and parents associations were members of the working party. It was chaired by Professor F. Vorst, emeritus professor of health care at the University of Limburg. The method was analogous to that of a comparable project relating to Child Health Surveillance, which was completed in England in

1989 (Hall, 1989). Several experts who were involved in the British project advised the Dutch working party in certain areas.

In five working conferences, the Dutch working party investigated the above-mentioned matters with respect to Child Health Care. By means of extensive international comparative literature studies, these conferences were prepared by a project team from the Centre for Research and Development of Youth Health Care and Youth Social Work of the University of Utrecht. On the basis of the literature studies, consensus meetings were held concerning the following subjects: the objectives of the Child Health Care system, immunizations, phenylketonuria (PKU) and congenital hypothyroidism (CHT) screenings, hearing examinations, visual examinations, language/speech examinations, periodic medical examinations, prevention of psychosocial and educational problems, health education, activities aimed at influencing social and physical environmental factors, and, finally, the quality and the organization of the Child Health Care system. The final version of the report was established on the basis of repeated discussions by the working party and advice obtained externally.

The Integral Evaluation Project was an effort to provide the best possible survey of the effectiveness and quality of the Dutch Child Health Care system. On the basis of its results, a great many recommendations have been formulated which are aimed at improving quality and effectiveness where possible. In addition, the project group has initiated a number of research programmes, with the aid of which further insight will be gained in the short term into effectiveness data which are not available as yet. In particular the instrument for the determination of cost-effectiveness ratios in the Child Health Care system, which will be developed by the Erasmus University, must be considered an important improvement. The most remarkable conclusion of the project is that the Dutch Child Health Care system may be considered a very solid kind of organized programmed prevention. The system owes its strength to its thorough national organization, and its firm establishment at community and district levels. The great trust this form of preventive care enjoys with the public is an essential precondition for an invariably high population coverage, which in its turn is responsible for the high degree of health benefit that is obtained with the system. The fact that there is room for improvement on many points does not detract from this conclusion. On the contrary, the possibility of such critical reflection on its own professional practice in this sector may serve as an example to many other health care sectors.

Reference

Hall, D.M.B. et al. (ed.) *Health for All Children*. A programme for Child Health Surveillance, New York 1989.

1 Aims, procedures and outcome measurement in pre-school Child Health Care

Outcome measurement in health care is practically always aimed at determining the outcome of separate interventions, whether these are of a preventive or curative nature. Think for instance of the studies into the effects of screening programmes for breast and cervical cancer, effects of heart transplants, or of information campaigns to influence smoking habits. Conversely there are few, if any, examples of studies into the effects of comprehensive and complex systems of care, such as pre-school Child Health Care. In comparison, one could, in this connection, think of outcome measurements of 'the' General Practice, or of 'the' Ambulatory Mental Health Care.

Outcome measurement of a system of care differs considerably in many respects from the evaluation of a single intervention. In studying the outcome of a system of care, multiple objectives as well as a whole range of intervention methods, and consequently a great diversity of outcome measures, have to be taken into account. Moreover, in evaluating a system of care, the possible connection or interference of the various constituent parts must be considered; in a system the whole is more than the sum of the parts. Owing to this complexity, outcome measurement of a system of care will necessarily have the character of a 'programme evaluation': a series of connected outcome studies, projected in time, the individual results of which may have implications for several parts of the system. Next to the study into the outcomes of its individual components, a programme evaluation also aims at providing insight into the overall effect of the system of care. In this way any duplications, prioritizations and gaps in the provision of care become apparent as well as aspects of organization, quality control and staffing policy.

In this chapter, the framework for the substance of such a programme evaluation of pre-school Child Health Care is sketched, starting with a description of the objectives. On the basis of the so-called ecological health model, used by the World Health Organization in the international programme 'Health for All by the Year 2000', a broad objective for pre-school Child Health Care is formulated. Subsequently, subsidiary objectives that can be made operational are derived from this. Then the operating procedures serving to attain these specific objectives are described. Finally the way to chart the effects of these procedures, related to the objectives, is explained.

1.1 Aims of pre-school Child Health Care

What then, exactly, are the aims and functions of pre-school Child Health Care? To begin with these do not, of course, constitute a static whole. At the time the first Child Health Clinics were established, some 100 years ago, the health of children was far worse than it is now. Because of poverty, ignorance of essential hygiene and lack of facilities, rampant infectious diseases and so on, infant mortality was very high (25% on average). Obviously, the main objective of 'Child Health Care' then was to fight such evils. The means used included social action, collective and individual education of mothers, the distribution of good quality milk and the opening of Child Health Clinics. As mortality and morbidity (from infectious diseases) decreased, the objectives of Child Health Care shifted. Gradually child development and 'mental hygiene' came into view as objects of care.

The main aim of pre-school Child Health Care, as expressed in 1972 by the Netherlands League of Maternity Care and Child Health Hygiene (Nederlandse Bond van Moederschapszorg en Kinderhygiene) was 'the promotion and safeguarding of the health, growth and development of young people'. In 1985 the Dutch Association of Child Health Care (Nederlandse Vereniging voor Jeugdgezondheidszorg) widened the aim: 'Child Health Care, within the welfare and health care system, aims to provide the longitudinal socio-medical guidance that will enable each individual, as a young person and as an adult, to function at his/her best individually and in a social context'. In the last few years, finally, a case has been argued for making more room within the system of care for the parents' responsibility for and contribution to the health and development of their children, as well as for considering the living environment of the child and its parents an object of Child Health Care.[1]

These ideas link up with the 'ecological health model', used by the WHO in realizing its aim 'Health for All by the Year 2000', and which in the Netherlands served as the basis for the Memorandum 2000 (Nota 2000). In the model, health is defined as 'a situation of equilibrium determined by the circumstances in which people are placed and the capacity they possess, or can acquire with the help of others, to defend themselves against disturbances' (Ministry of Welfare, Public Health and Cultural Affairs

---

[1]See e.g. De Winter (1990).

1986). Four groups of health determinants are mentioned: physical factors; health behaviour; social and physical environment; and the system of care itself. A health problem (collective or individual) may arise through the interaction of the various determinants. Specific health objectives (targets) must therefore be pursued by influencing all relevant health determinants.

From this perspective the aim of pre-school Child Health Care can now be defined as follows: 'The promotion and safeguarding of a healthy physical, mental and social development of the population of pre-school children, starting from the parents' personal responsibility, by means of influencing the relevant health determinants, namely physical factors, health behaviour and relevant environmental factors, including the system of care itself'.

This general aim can be translated into four subsidiary objectives that can be made operational.

- It is the objective of pre-school Child Health Care to improve immunity against infectious diseases.

- It is the objective of pre-school Child Health Care to detect the threat of individual health risks and disorders in time and, if necessary, refer.

- It is the objective of pre-school Child Health Care to promote, at an individual and collective level, the personal competence and the responsibility of parents with regard to their children, if necessary by advancing their understanding of the health condition and (potential) development of their child and by increasing their competence (health promoting behaviour).

- It is the objective of pre-school Child Health Care to provide insight into the health condition of (groups of) young people, to point out social risk factors that threaten health and to contribute to the elimination of such factors.

1.2 Procedures in pre-school Child Health Care

Obviously it is the task of pre-school Child Health Care so to shape its procedures (in connection with other organizations) that the above objectives can be optimally realized. If the extent to which these objectives are attained is to be determined, the methods to do so must be established. These methods, after all, are the means by which the ends have to be reached. It will then be possible to measure outcome for each method used and also for the system of care as a whole. The latter measurement can only be an approximation: in the first place pre-school Child Health Care is not the only active factor (wide variables such as prosperity also influence the state of health), and in the second place the effect of the aggregate of methods does not equal the sum of the parts. One important reason for this is that the methods at the service of pre-school Child Health Care are not at all of equal order. On the one hand, for instance there are specific, unambiguous interventions such as immunizations and screenings that serve a well defined health target; on the other hand there are activities with a much wider scope, such as counselling or giving advice and information on the development of children and so on. Finally the presence, accessibility and social roots of the system of care are major preconditions themselves. However effective specific methods (such as immunization) are, if there is no good organization for reaching the population the effect on health will be considerably reduced. An adequate organization of the system itself, in other words, is a necessary condition for the effectiveness of the whole of pre-school Child Health Care.

Therefore, if we are to chart pre-school Child Health Care, two levels should be distinguished. The first level is the provision of the required conditions: the organized system of care, the extensive network of clinics for babies and young children, from which numerous preventive and health promotion activities are developed. Pre-school Child Health Care is carried out by nurses and Medical Clinical Officers in clinics, in homes and for groups. Support is given by District Medical Officers and Senior Nurses as well as by educational experts, dieticians and health education consultants, in their specific fields. The second level consists of the specific medical, nursing and educational methods for prevention and intervention, including immunization, screenings, counselling and the drawing up of health profiles. These two levels are considered below.

1.2.1 The organized system of care

For decades, pre-school preventive health care in the Netherlands has been carried out by the 'Cross' organizations.[2] Amsterdam, where this care is provided by the Municipal Health Service, is an exception to the rule. Pre-

---

[2]For a long time 'Cross Associations' (Kruisverenigingen) have been active in the Netherlands in the fields of social and preventive medicine and home nursing on behalf of their members as well as of the general public. The National Cross Association (National Kruisvereniging) represented the regional cross associations at national level. In 1990 the National Cross Association merged with the National Council for Home Help (Centrale Raad voor de Gezinsverzorging) to form the National Association for Community Nursing and Home Care (Landelijke Vereniging voor Thuiszorg), established at Bunnik. In this book the regional organizations will be referred to as 'Community Health Care'.

school Child Health Care takes place in a number of different ways: in Child Health Clinics, in home visits, group education and 'external' activities including participation in working groups on Early Detection and in neighbourhood networks for youth welfare work. In the course of years, a very close national network for pre-school Child Health Care has been built up through local organizations. Both the population and the authorities consider the clinics and the connected activities as a basic facility; practically every parent in the Netherlands made and makes regular use of them. The basic character of this facility can also be seen from the way it is financed: pre-school Child Health Care is largely paid for under the Exceptional Medical Expenses Act (Algemene Wet op de Bijzondere Ziektekosten AWBZ), which makes this form of care accessible to everyone and thus provides a nationwide guaranteed basic package. Coverage figures are an extremely important criterion for assessing the adequate functioning of such basic preventive care. A high population coverage is after all a *conditio sine qua non* for the performance of practically all functions concerned with the aims described in section 1.1. For many years now the coverage of pre-school Child Health Care has been accurately recorded. The baby clinics have a stable coverage of over 95%, the clinics for pre-school children some 85%. PKU/CHT screening covers 99.6%, the immunization level is more than 93% (Drewes 1989), and the range of hearing screening by the Ewing method is 86% (NSDSK 1989)[3]. No percentages are known of the number of home visits made annually by district nurses, but they are estimated at one million per year (Bos & De Winter 1989). International comparison shows that, certainly as far as immunizations, PKU/CHT screening and hearing screening are concerned, these figures are among the highest in the world. Partly for these reasons, the Netherlands has the lowest child mortality among the under-fives in the world after Japan, Sweden and Finland.

Another important criterion for assessing the Dutch system of Child Health Care is the quality of the system and its reaction speed. Health and health care are not static. The health situation of the population in care changes, old threats lessen and new risks may present themselves. Scientific opinions change, making new forms of intervention possible. For this reason the system of care should possess some degree of flexibility and the ability to meet new challenges with new methods. In the past few years the effectiveness of a soundly organized and flexibly operating pre-school Child Health Care has been demonstrated several times. One example of this is the introduction of a new vaccination against measles, mumps and rubella (MMR) a few years ago, which, within a year of its introduction, achieved the same high degree of immunization of over 90% as the long established

---

[3]The majority of the remaining children have their hearing screened by other methods. See Chapter 4, footnote 3.

immunizations of the National Immunization Programme (Rijksvaccinatie Programma RVP)[4]. Another example concerns health education: by changing the advice about laying babies on their stomachs a quick and sharp decrease in the incidence of cot death was brought about (De Jonge 1992).

As stated above, high coverage as well as the capacity to react quickly and adequately to new health risks or new points of view should be considered necessary conditions for adequate functioning of pre-school Child Health Care. The positive score on these criteria can therefore be considered an important outcome of Dutch pre-school Child Health Care.

1.2.2 Methods of intervention and prevention

Different criteria are used to classify prevention. Firstly, a distinction is often made between health promotion, health protection and prevention of sickness. The second well-known distinction, between primary, secondary and tertiary prevention, mainly refers to the stage in the course of the sickness or disorder at the moment of preventive intervention. Thirdly, a distinction is usually made between collective and individual prevention, in order to indicate whether the prevention addresses the population, or groups of it, or the needs of individuals. Each of these classifications has serious shortcomings for the description and evaluation of pre-school Child Health Care. Many activities undertaken in this connection aim, for instance, at health promotion as well as at prevention of sickness, or they make smooth transitions between primary, secondary and tertiary prevention. The distinction between collective and individual prevention also causes a lot of confusion, since collective prevention is often carried out individually and individual prevention may also have a collective significance.

Finally, in a recent recommendation, the National Health Council (Nationale Raad voor de Volksgezondheid NRV) focused attention on the notion of 'programmed prevention'.[5] Programmed prevention is described as: 'systematically executed preventive activities carried out according to a fixed division of tasks and procedure and aimed at a defined target group, the coverage of the target group being monitored' (Van de Water & Davidse 1992). With regard to the implementation, a distinction is made

---

[4]See Chapter 2.

[5]This NRV recommendation is partly based on a preliminary report called *Organizational strengthening of prevention in primary care (Organisatiorische versterking van preventie in de eerstelijnszorg)*, published by NIPG/TNO, Leiden (Van de Water & Davidse 1992).

between programmes with an individual and those with a collective approach: 'a programme that requires individual targeting is called individual targeted programmed prevention and programmes that entail collective execution are called collective prevention programmes' (National Health Council 1992). With respect to Child Health Care, a third category could be added, namely group targeted prevention programmes (such as group education or group clinics). Pre-school Child Health Care in its entirety may be described as a mainly individually targeted form of organized programmed prevention. Collectively, targeted programmed prevention mainly takes place outside the sector's field of responsibility. The mass media campaigns for the prevention of caries, child abuse and accidents are examples.

The practical activities of pre-school Child Health Care may be divided, within the framework of individually targeted programmed prevention, into two categories, namely standardized prevention programmes and prevention programmes geared to the individual characteristics and needs of parent and child. In this report the latter category will be referred to as 'prevention to measure' (or individually geared 'prevention'). Examples of standardized prevention programmes are: the National Immunization Programme; PKU and CHT screening; hearing screening; checks for visual disorders; developmental surveillance; detection of language and speech disorders; as well as some types of health education (for instance Accident Prevention Cards)[6]. Examples of parts of programmes that require specific individual gearing (prevention to measure) are individual education, guidance and counselling on the subjects of development, care, food and education. Finally there are parts of programmes which are in the process of being further standardized, such as the Periodical Health Examination[7].

The application of the 'ecological health model', as already described, implies that the main aims of pre-school Child Health Care, the promotion and protection of the health and development of young children, are to be realized by influencing the relevant health determinants. Pre-school Child Health Care has a number of methods at its disposal for this purpose. They are classified here in two ways. In the first place a functional classification is used, based on the subsidiary objectives of pre-school Child Health Care described in section 1.1. This classification makes it possible on the one hand to chart the relationships between ends and means systematically, and

---

[6]Accident Prevention Cards are a tool to promote safety; accidents being the major cause of death in children. Each card contains safety information aimed at a specific age group. They are handed out at Child Health Clinics to make parents aware of accident risks at specific stages of development of the child. This helps parents to take safety measures in time.

[7]Proposals for the standardized recording of the Periodical Health Examination have in the meantime been worked out: see Chapter 8 of this report.

on the other hand to consider any gaps in the delivery of care. In the second place a classification is made with the help of the concepts of standardized prevention (SP) and prevention to measure (MP)[8]. Thus the following overview is arrived at:

a   Subs.obj.:   Immunity against major infectious diseases.
    Method: (SP) National Vaccination Programme.
b   Subs.obj.:   Detecting and identifying individual risk factors
                  and disorders.
    Methods: (MP) Periodical Health Examination (if recorded: SP,
                  see Chapter 8).
                  (SP) Screenings (PKU/CHT, hearing, vision).
                  (SP) Recorded Early Detection methods (Van Wiechen
                  check-list[9], ED language instrument).
c   Subs.obj.:   Promoting parental understanding and competence
                  through education (collective and individual),
                  counselling and guidance.
    Methods: (MP) Ascertaining demand for support and
                  information.
                  (MP) Individual guidance, education and counselling
                  (for instance as a result of examinations listed under
                  b above).
                  (SP) Group education (for instance with regard to
                  teaching subjects).
                  (SP) Printed information (by means of the Growth
                  Book, Toddler Information Leaflets[10], Accident
                  Prevention Cards and so on).
                  (SP) Possible introduction of a parent-held record
                  (Child Health Care record in the possession of
                  parents).

------

[8]It should be noted with regard to the classification into standardized and individually targeted parts that this is a broad classification: in practice standardized components are accompanied by individually targeted elements. A well known example is the extra individual attention that has to be given to motivate some parents to take part in the immunization programme.

[9]Partly based on the Denver Developmental Scale, the 'Van Wiechen' check-list was developed in the early eighties to promote the systematic examination of development (motor development, language and speech, personality and social behaviour) and to achieve uniform national registration. For details see Chapter 6, section 5.

[10]The 'Growth Book' has been issued to all parents of new-born babies in the Netherlands since 1978. It aims to give the parents the information to help them care for and raise their children. For further details see section 10.1.2. Toddler Information Leaflets are folders with age-specific information on the development of the child. Subjects include: eating, sleeping, play, behaviour, toilet training, obstinacy.

d   Subs.obj.:   Pointing out health-threatening risk factors in the social and physical environment.

    Methods: (SP) Systematic registration of the condition of the health of (groups of) children; drawing up health profiles.
(MP and SP) Identifying and if possible influencing factors in the surroundings that threaten health and development, such as environmental dangers, neighbourhood safety (including safety in traffic, lack of play opportunities and so on).
(MP and SP) Identifying groups of children that run extraordinary risks (owing to an accumulation of individual and social risk factors, for instance).

If the promotion of an adequately functioning system of care is considered to be a major precondition for achieving the above objectives (or, as in the ecological health model, a 'health determinant'), more methods can be specified which satisfy these preconditions. For instance, participation in cooperative bodies and in neighbourhood networks, maintaining a quality control and monitoring system, organizational adaptations and so on.

In day-to-day pre-school Child Health Care practice the above activities are generally carried out in conjunction with one another. Because various determinants may be involved, various methods are indicated, based on an actual health target. Two examples may illustrate this.

Example 1: Nutrition

Target: Promoting and safeguarding a good nutritional condition

Methods: • Physical examination of nutritional condition

           • Information on age-linked nutritional needs and nutritional habits (standardized or individually geared health education)

           • Indication of risk factors at population level with regard to nutrition (PCBs in breast milk for instance)

           • Optimizing counselling opportunities (such as by dieticians).

Example 2: Psychomotor development

Target: Promoting and safeguarding optimum psychomotor development

Methods: • Early detection (Van Wiechen check-list)

           • Education on stages of development (health education, Growth Book)

           • Optimizing a system of referral of detected disorders.

1.3 Outcome measurement

For a number of reasons the determination of the outcome of pre-school Child Health Care is not a simple and unambiguous matter. The first problem is that the outcome of prevention often becomes visible only in the long run. This means that the outcome of pre-school Child Health Care could in fact chiefly be shown through longitudinal and therefore very costly research. A timely referral in connection with a suspected developmental disorder for instance, is an important, but by no means isolated outcome measure. The ultimate effect should be a decrease in the number of people suffering from developmental disorders or their results.

This immediately gives rise to a second problem, namely the question of how far or to what extent the effects obtained can actually be attributed to pre-school Child Health Care. This is difficult, because quite a number of other variables are involved, such as general prosperity and hygiene, or the reliability and effectiveness of diagnosis and treatment that take place outside the pre-school Child Health Care service. In other words, if long-term outcome measures were to be used it would hardly be possible to discern which outcomes actually result from Child Health Care activities. A third problem is posed by the broad, differentiated aims of pre-school Child Health Care, as set out in the previous section. Especially the fact that this service is not only concerned with the prevention of unequivocal illnesses or disorders, but also with such complex problem areas as psycho-social development and teaching relationships. This results in the need to apply an equally differentiated range of standardized and individually targeted methods. This again gives rise to the problem that the outcome measurement of programmed prevention is usually simpler to realize than that of prevention to measure. Not only does systematic data recording take place (in pre-school Child Health Care as well) with regard to such standardized programmes but, for instance with regard to the evaluation of screening programmes, there is also an extensive system of epidemiological and statistical concepts available. The outcomes of prevention to measure, on the other hand, are rather more difficult to depict, because of the different character of the interventions for each individual situation and the connected problems for systematic recording.

Other methodological and technical problems for the ascertaining of pre-school Child Health Care outcomes are:

- The absence of control groups. Just because of the practically complete coverage of the population it is not really possible to decide what the outcomes would be of 'no prevention'.

- Pre-school Child Health Care not only focuses on 'health benefits', but is also aimed at enhancing the quality of life. The question is in how far this can be measured by the QUALY method (quality-adjusted life-years).

- The occurrence of various forms of distortion when ascertaining the outcomes of screening (lead-time bias, length bias, self-selection bias and overdiagnosis bias).

As argued in the introduction to this report, the Integral Evaluation Child Health Care project was aimed in the first place at gaining insight into existing data on cost effectiveness of parts of pre-school Child Health Care. For this purpose a number of literature searches have been made and included in this report.

In the course of the project however, the conclusion was reached that a specific set of instruments should be developed for a permanent and comprehensive insight into the cost-effectiveness ratios within pre-school Child Health Care. The Institute for Social Health Care (Instituut voor Maatschappelijke Gezondheidszorg) of the Erasmus University of Rotterdam was commissioned to undertake this. In the research project the outcomes and costs of screening methods will be reviewed first, based on the following broad definition of the concept of screening: 'when (at fixed times and according to a fixed protocol) parents are asked questions and observations are being carried out on children to ascertain whether a number of defined health disorders (a) are probably present or threaten to arise and/or (b) further diagnosis and/or therapy is needed, it may be said that screening takes place for this series of defined disorders' (Van der Maas 1991). According to Van der Maas, the outcomes of screening fall into two main groups: bringing forward diagnosis and the health benefits achieved by this. Once data are available with regard to the effectiveness of parts of pre-school Child Health Care it is possible, in principle, to start determining the ratio of cost and effectiveness. The 'cost' of pre-school Child Health Care should include the collective means employed to maintain clinics and so on, as well as the outlay for the training and refresher courses of staff, and the costs incurred in the follow-up work of pre-school Child Health Care. After all, when a diagnosis is made by specific Early Detection activities, costs are generated in the diagnostic and treatment circuit. On the other hand there are a number of savings: some costs do not arise because other provisions (for instance more expensive treatment) are not needed as a result of activities within pre-school Child Health Care. Taking the matter even further, there may also be savings because disablement, for instance, can be prevented. In this way, cost profiles can be calculated for each part of pre-school Child Health Care. An estimate of the ratio of costs and effectiveness of pre-school Child Health Care thus becomes feasible. The instrument to be developed by Erasmus

University is being tested on hearing screening by the Ewing method and on the new Early Detection language tool. The first results are presented in this report. In the long run it is intended to analyse all appropriate parts of pre-school Child Health Care.

1.4 The structure of the report

The following steps have so far been taken for the purpose of outcome measurement:

- a main aim was formulated

- four subsidiary objectives that can be made operational were derived from this

- a number of standardized and individually targeted prevention programmes were organized around these subsidiary objectives.

Within the framework of the present project a number of international literature searches were made for effectiveness data of separate components of the programme of care. In this first stage of the project emphasis has been placed on standardized components. The outcomes of these were expected to be easiest to chart. Such prevention programmes are usually preceded by scientific research and careful recording and monitoring of them will also take place. A second argument to give priority to the evaluation of standardized components is of an ethical nature: as against prevention to measure, where activities are initiated within the framework of an 'interview' between parent and professional, standardized components more or less imply 'unsolicited' delivery by professionals. There is an even greater need for scientific justification in such cases (Van de Water & Davidse 1992).

In Chapters 2 to 7 these standardized components are dealt with. They are immunizations, PKU/CHT screening, hearing screening, early detection of vision disorders, developmental surveillance and the detection of speech and language disorders.

The central questions of the separate studies are:
- What are the target problems?
- What is known of the aetiology and the (natural) course?
- What figures on incidence and prevalence are available with regard to the target problems?
- What methods of prevention or intervention are available?

- What are the relevant outcome measures?
- What data are available (internationally) on the effectiveness of the various methods?
- Is additional outcome assessment necessary?

In the course of the project sufficient particulars with regard to a number of subjects were found to be available. Several literature searches however led to the conclusion that supplementary research was required. Authoritative institutes have already drawn up research proposals.

Chapters 8, 9 and 10 deal with elements that so far have wholly or partly the character of 'prevention to measure'. They are the Periodical Health Examination (PHE), the prevention of psycho-social and teaching problems, and health education. Whether certain activities may be suitable for a more standardized approach is examined.

Chapter 11 has a somewhat different character. It deals with aspects that in fact play an important part in pre-school Child Health Care, but have not until now, been considered very explicitly. These are activities targeted at influencing the health determinants 'social and physical environment' and the 'system of care'. Chapter 11 considers how a contribution can be made from pre-school Child Health Care to the detection of and intervention in health threatening factors originating from the social and physical environment. It is shown that extra stimulus should be given to cooperation with organizations in the fields of health care, youth welfare work, day care and education as well as with municipal authorities.

Finally this report gives a summary of conclusions and recommendations.

References

Bos, M.W. & Winter, M. de: Het consultatiebureau is niet van gisteren, in: Bos, M.W. & Winter, M. de (red.): *Jeugdgezondheidszorg in de toekomst*, Lisse: Swets en Zeitlinger, 1989, pp.7–13.

Drewes, J.: Kwaliteitsbewaking in de jeugdgezondheidszorg, in: Bos, M.W. & Winter, M. de (red.): *Jeugdgezondheidszorg in de toekomst*, Lisse: Swets en Zeitlinger, 1989, pp.89–104.

Jonge, G.J. de: Wiegedood in Nederland 1985–1990, *Tijdschrift voor Jeugdgezondheidszorg* 24 (1992) 1, 3–6.

Maas, P.J. van der: Kosten-effectiviteits-vraagstellingen in de jeugdge-zondheidszorg, *Tijdschrift voor Jeugdgezondheidszorg* 23 (1991) 3, 45–46.

Ministerie van WVC: *Over de ontwikkeling van het gezondheidsbeleid: feiten, beschouwingen en beleidsvoornemens (Nota 2000)*, Den Haag: Sdu, 1986.

NSDSK (Nederlandse Stichting voor het Dove en Slechthorende Kind): *Jaarverslag VOG*, Amsterdam 1989.

NRV (Nationale Raad voor de Volksgezondheid): *Advies inzake versterking van de preventie in de eerstelijnszorg*, publ.nr. 6/92, Zoetermeer: NRV, 1992.

Water, H.P.A. van de & Davidse, W.: *Organisatorische versterking van preventie in de eerstelijns gezondheidszorg. Tweede pre-advies ten behoeve van het door de Staatssecretaris van WVC aan de Nationale Raad voor de Volksgezondheid gevraagde advies inzake het preventiebeleid in Nederland*, publ.nr. 92.008, Leiden: NIPG/TNO, 1992.

Winter, M. de: *De kwaliteit van het kinderlijk bestaan*, Bunnik 1990 (oratie).

Further reading

Lim-Feyen, J.F.: Doelstellingen in de preventieve jeugdgezondheidszorg, *Medisch Contact* 43 (1988) 44, 1357.

Nederlandse Bond voor Moederschapszorg en Kinderhygiëne: *Jeugdgezond-heidszorg: inhoud en taakuitvoering*, Utrecht 1972.

NVJG (Nederlandse Vereniging voor Jeugdgezondheidszorg): *Functie- en taak-omschrijving van een jeugdarts in een jeugdgezondheidszorgteam*, Utrecht 1985.

NVJG: *De Jeugdgezondheidszorg in 2000; beleidsplan 1990*, Utrecht 1990.

Unicef: *The State of the World's Children*, Oxford 1991.

2 Immunizations

Internationally, the Netherlands has a name for its excellent prevention of infectious diseases, resulting from a very high immunization uptake. Since 1979, the national average for all immunizations has been more than 90% (GHI 1981a, 1991a, 1992). This has been accomplished thanks to excellent computerized administration, to a great willingness (virtually 100%) on the part of the public to make use of the National Immunization Programme (RVP)[1], to a well-developed and easily accessible network of Child Health Clinics and the Child Health Care Departments of the District and Municipal Health Services (GGD). The infectious diseases against which the population has been systematically immunized have practically disappeared in the Netherlands, except in some communities where there is a concentration of people who, for ideological or religious reasons, refuse to have their children immunized.

In this chapter, the scientific foundations of immunization in the Netherlands are reviewed. The original Dutch text has been updated for this English edition, in which the situation as of September 1993 is described. To put things into perspective, the RVP and the way it is organized are outlined, followed by a synopsis of the immunization programmes. For reasons of brevity, the diseases are not described in detail. The reader is referred to textbooks (for example Avery et al. 1989, Ball & Gray 1984 and, in Dutch, Stoop & Vossen 1990). Finally, the costs, effectiveness, benefits, and the relationship between these three, are discussed.

2.1 The National Immunization Programme (RVP)

Each year, the Minister for Welfare, Public Health and Cultural Affairs (WVC) lays down the RVP for that year on the recommendations of the National Health Council (Nationale Raad voor de Volksgezondheid NRV),

---

[1]The National Immunization Programme is referred to further in this chapter by the acronym RVP

having listened to the recommendations of the Chief Medical Inspector (Geneeskundige Hoofdinspecteur GHI), the Director-General of the National Institute of Public Health and Environmental Protection (Rijksinstituut voor Volksgezondheid en Milieuhygiëne RIVM) and the Health Insurance Board (Ziekenfondsraad). Each year the Inspectorate publishes a leaflet setting out the immunization programme for that year, and distributes this among the officials responsible for implementation. The Inspectorate sees to it that the RVP is carried out in accordance with the annual programme. Only the vaccines listed in Table 1 can be provided within the framework of the RVP; other immunizations fall outside its coverage. The immunizations of the RVP have not always been the same: adjustments are made from time to time as a result of new epidemiological insights and technical possibilities.

The initial impetus for the RVP was the polio epidemic in 1956 which claimed 2206 victims. A diphtheria-pertussis-tetanus vaccine (DPT) had been available in the Netherlands since 1952, and was extensively used in the child health clinics, so that 70% of the children had been immunized with DPT by the time (1957) the RVP was introduced (Hannik 1963). At an even earlier stage, children in the Netherlands were being immunized against smallpox and diphtheria. With the introduction of the RVP in 1957, inactivated triple polio vaccine (Salk vaccine) was used, initially as a separate polio vaccine and from 1962 onwards as a combined diphtheria-tetanus-pertussis-polio vaccine. This has continued to the present day. The use of the Salk vaccine makes the Netherlands fairly exceptional because in most other countries live oral polio vaccine (Sabin vaccine) is used. The latter is only used in the Netherlands in cases of polio outbreaks. The situation in the Netherlands differs from that in other countries (geographically, demographically, logistically and financially) and because of this the advantages and disadvantages of using the two vaccines are weighed up differently in this country than elsewhere (Dutch National Health Council; see: Gezondheidsraad 1982b).

In 1974, the immunization of 11-year-old girls against rubella (German measles) was started as a separate immunization, followed by a separate immunization against measles in 1976. In 1987, both disappeared again from the RVP with the introduction of the combined immunization against mumps, measles and rubella (MMR). Within the scope of the RVP, it is possible to immunize against measles and rubella only by means of the MMR-vaccine. On 1 April 1993, the immunization against *Haemophilus Influenzae type b* was added to the RVP. This will not necessarily mark the end of the list of diseases against which prevention can be offered in the form of immunization (Ruitenberg et al. 1984, Huisman 1985, Ruitenberg 1989). However, before any further additions are made, it must be quite clear that the practicability of the programme will not be jeopardized, and that the motivation of parents and professionals will not diminish as a result (Bijkerk 1986a). In the countries that surround the Netherlands, and certainly in developing countries, different immunization schedules are used. The case is argued that national immunization programmes should be harmonized. In principle, the only differences allowed should be those based on solid scientific (epidemiological and serological) foundations. However, logistic and financial limitations also contribute to the ultimate form of the schedule (Bijkerk 1986b). The RVP for 1993 is shown in Table 1.

Table 1 National Immunization Programme (RVP) in the Netherlands 1993

Immunization(s)	(Dutch)	age
DPT/Polio-1 + Hib-1	(DKTP-1 + Hib-1)	3 months
DPT/Polio-2 + Hib-2	(DKTP-2 + Hib-2)	4 months
DPT/Polio-3 + Hib-3	(DKTP-3 + Hib-3)	5 months
DPT/Polio-4 + Hib-4	(DKTP-4 + Hib-4)	11 months
MMR-1	(BMR-1)	14 months
DT/Polio-5	(DTP-5)	4 years
DT/Polio-6 + MMR-2	(DTP-6 + BMR-2)	9 years

D = Diphtheria	D = Diphtheria
P = Pertussis	K = Pertussis (kinkhoest)
T = Tetanus	T = Tetanus
Polio	P = Polio
M = Mumps	B = Mumps (bof)
M = Measles	M = Measles (mazelen)
R = Rubella	R = Rubella (rodehond)

2.1.1 Implementation of the RVP

The RVP is implemented by the two Child Health Care systems in the Netherlands. The first are the Community Health Care Organizations, which are responsible for preventive health care services for pre-school children. From the moment children go to school, preventive health care is carried out by the departments of Child Health Care of the District and Municipal Health Authorities (GGD). These authorities also conduct campaigns for schoolchildren who, for some reason or other, have been incompletely, or not at all, immunized. Implementation of the RVP is the responsibility of the Provincial Immunization Administration (Provinciale Entadministratie PEA). Each PEA has appointed a qualified doctor (Consultant Community Paediatrician) who is responsible for the medical aspects of the RVP. Immunization is a medical procedure and therefore must be performed either by a doctor or under the supervision of a doctor. In the case of the RVP, these doctors work in the child health clinics or are school doctors. General practitioners and paediatricians are involved in the RVP to a limited extent, namely in cases where immunization involves a particular risk for a specific child or in cases where children are hospitalized. Immunization may, under certain conditions, be delegated to qualified nurses (Jefferson et al. 1987, LVT 1991).

The administrative organization has been assigned to the Provincial Immunization Adminstration PEA (Ministry of Public Health and Environmental Protection 1974a,b). The provinces of Overijssel and Flevoland share one PEA, the other 10 provinces have a PEA of their own, as do the cities of Amsterdam and Rotterdam, so that there are 13 PEAs in the country. In addition to the administrative organization of the RVP, the PEAs have also been charged with the administration of the screening programmes for phenylketonuria (PKU), congenital hypothyroidism (CHT) and of the combined screening and immunization programme for hepatitis B.

The vaccines for the RVP are procured by the PEAs from, or via, the RIVM. The PEAs take care of the distribution to the Child Health Clinics and the District and Municipal Health Services where the immunizations are given.

For the benefit of those responsible for implementation, details of the RVP are set out in guidelines, which were originally published by the Medical Inspectorate (GHI 1981b). Because these guidelines had never been updated, most child health clinics used a publication of the Overijssel and Flevoland PEA with practical guidelines and background information (Burgmeijer & Bolscher 1990). Recently, the information was updated and published in book form, together with useful information about other immunizations frequently given to children (Burgmeijer & Bolscher 1993).

2.1.2 Financing of the RVP

Since 1 January 1974, the RVP has been financed by the Exceptional Medical Expenses Act (Algemene Wet Bijzondere Ziektekosten AWBZ) (Ministry of Public Health and Environmental Protection 1974c). On the basis of this act, the implementation of the RVP was elaborated in a number of parliamentary decrees (Ministry of Public Health and Environmental Protection 1974a, 1977, 1981). As already mentioned, the Minister for Welfare, Public Health and Cultural Affairs lays down the immunization programme, which states which groups of insured persons qualify for immunization with the named vaccines. In special cases, the PEA can decide to administer RVP vaccinations to insured persons other than those who belong to the categories stated in the RVP (Ministry of Public Health and Environmental Protection 1974a). The processing and storage of data concerning the insured persons with respect to the RVP, up to and including the twelfth year of life, is carried out by the PEA. In practice this means that, within the framework of the RVP (and consequently financed in pursuance of the AWBZ), immunizations may be given up to the twelfth birthday.

2.2 Effects of immunization

Immunization can be regarded as the controlled stimulation of the immune system. A certain quantity and quality of pathogenic micro-organisms are administered at a predetermined moment, to ensure that the body reacts with an immune response, and, at the same time, to keep the risk of adverse reactions to an acceptable minimum. In other words, immunizations combine a very high level of effectiveness with a minimum of risk. The point of departure for all immunizations is that the risks involved must be much lower than the risks of undergoing 'wild infection'. The question of effectiveness has individual and epidemiological aspects. In addition to this, distinction should be made between positive and negative effects (Table 2).

Table 2   Positive and negative effects of immunizations at individual and population levels

Positive effect	Negative effect
Individual level	
● immune response	● no immune response
● preventing illness	● adverse reactions
	● costs caused by reactions
Population level	
● herd immunity	
● decreased mortality	
● decreased morbidity	
● savings on health care	

2.2.1 Effects at individual level

2.2.1.1 Immunity by seroconversion after immunization

The aim of immunization at the individual level is to achieve immunity. Proof that this effect has been produced can only be obtained by demonstrating specific antibodies (or a rise in antibody level). But the question of effectiveness cannot be fully answered simply by demonstrating a rise of antibodies, the following questions must be answered as well:

- How long will the specific antibodies last?

- Is the quality of the resistance after immunization equal to that obtained after undergoing 'wild infection'?

The chance that a good immune response will occur varies with the immunization. It is smallest in immunization against tuberculosis (BCG vaccination) at around 70%. For all other immunizations, it is at least 90% (Burgmeijer & Bolscher 1990, 1993). If no immune response occurs after immunization, this does not mean that the same will happen after an identical immunization. This is why the MMR immunization is administered twice (at 14 months and at 9 years), by which means, in addition to giving those with second thoughts a chance, a proportion of the 5% of children in whom no immune response occurred the first time, are still protected. When an immune response occurs after immunization with live vaccine, as a rule no further immunization is necessary. On the other hand, inactivated vaccines require a series of immunizations to obtain the desired level of antibodies.

In choosing the age at which immunization can best be given, a number of (sometimes contradictory) factors play a role. Consequently, a good choice can never be more than the best compromise. On the one hand, a child will preferably not be immunized if a sufficient titre of maternal antibodies can be demonstrated. Of course, this only applies for diseases the antibodies to which can pass through the placenta. On the other hand, it is desirable that the child be immunized as soon as possible against diseases the antibodies to which cannot pass through the placenta. In the first case, it is desirable for immunization to be postponed until about the age of 3–6 months; in the second case immunization should take place as soon as possible after birth. Age to some extent determines the developmental stage of the immune system. However, its influence has long been overestimated and these days no adjustment is made for prematurity (Verbrugge 1986).

The period during which immunization offers protection varies with the disease. A relatively short period of protection (10–15 years) is obtained after BCG, diphtheria and tetanus vaccination. Medium to long term immunity (approximately 35 years) is obtained after rubella immunization. Immunizations against polio, mumps and measles probably offer life-long protection. The duration of the protection of a whooping cough immunization is not known exactly, but is, in any case, sufficiently long to offer protection during infancy and early childhood. In some cases a wild infection provides more prolonged protection than immunization. For this reason some doctors and nurses erroneously discourage immunization. Discouraging immunizations in the belief that 'children in our protective society are better off if they undergo the diseases of childhood in the normal way' (some people even consider this to be a right) suggests an unprofessional attitude that unnecessarily exposes children to greater risks (Van der Stel 1986).

In all cases (tetanus excepted) the length of protection offered by immunization meets the target set. Life-long protection against rubella is not necessary for the protection of the individual. On the individual level the aim is to protect the woman in the reproductive period. However, from the point of view of public health it can be very important to have a rubella immunization that produces life-long immunity, because in that case it will be possible to stop the circulation of the virus in the population (De Boo et al. 1986). It is worth bearing in mind that there are also diseases in which a wild infection offers no protection at all (tetanus), or only partial protection (polio, depending on the type of virus).

The effectiveness of immunization may also depend on whether or not a re-immunization is given. After a single whooping cough immunization the vaccine efficacy is 59%, and after two re-immunizations this builds up to 66% and 95% respectively (Bijkerk 1986a). It is because of this phenomenon that, for children who have not been immunized or have been immunized incompletely, there is a special schedule aimed at achieving so called basic immunization after which, depending on its age, the child qualifies for regular RVP immunizations (Burgmeijer & Bolscher 1990, 1993).

2.2.1.2 Side effects

Even when the RVP is implemented in accordance with the most stringent guidelines, from the production of the vaccine to the injection, there is still a risk of adverse reactions following immunization. Reactions to immunization can be classified according to degree, extent, type of vaccine, and the moment at which they occur (Burgmeijer & Bolscher 1993). Doctors are urged to report major and unexpected reactions to the Medical Centre for Immunizations (Medisch Centrum Immunisaties MCI) of the RIVM, which then launches an investigation. The National Health Council (Nationale Raad voor de

Volksgezondheid) reports annually on the findings of the MCI (Dutch National Health Council; see: Gezondheidsraad 1972, 1986, 1987, 1988, 1989, 1990).

Each year, more than 2 million immunizations are carried out within the framework of the RVP. In 1990, 99 major reactions were reported, 84 of which were reported following DPT/polio immunizations, two after simultaneous immunization with DPT/polio and MMR, and 13 after measles immunization. In 1990 no side effects of Hib immunizations were reported. The Committee on Side Effects of Vaccines (Commissie Bijwerkingen Vaccins) of the National Health Council considered the causal relationship between immunization and reaction convincing in 86 cases, probable in four cases, and possible in nine cases. The most frequent side effects were collapse and local major reactions after DPT/polio-1 (23 and 10 cases, respectively), and convulsions after DPT/polio-4 (12 cases). Only two cases of encephalitis, and one anaphylactic reaction were reported. Collapse occurred particularly after DTP/polio-1, that is among the category of youngest children. Convulsions occurred particularly after DPT/polio-4 and the MMR-1 immunizations. In 1990, the Committee received 10 reports of deaths that were thought to be associated with immunizations that had been given several days or weeks earlier. In one case the report could not be assessed, in six cases the connection was considered improbable, in one case possible and in two cases convincing. These latter two cases concerned children who, 8 days after a MMR immunization, had developed status epilepticus which resulted in death. However, both children had serious metabolic disorders, were susceptible to infections and had food intolerances. They had been given DPT/polio immunizations after careful consideration, and these had not caused any problems (Dutch National Health Council; see Gezondheidsraad) 1991).

In England, a National Childhood Encephalopathy Study (NCES) was carried out in the period 1976–1979 in which the risk of serious, but transitory neurological complications following DPT immunization was estimated at 1:140,000 while the chance of permanent brain damage was estimated at 1:330,000 (Miller et al. 1981). This is considerably higher than the above mentioned number of reports in the Netherlands. However, the NCES has been criticized over the years and the results of this study are no longer considered valid (ACIP 1991). Major reactions following DPT/polio immunizations can, without any doubt, be attributed exclusively to the P-component (Hannik 1984, 1985), and can be traced to the nature of the vaccine (killed *Bordetella pertussis* bacteria). Although research has been done in Japan and Sweden on an acellular vaccine (Sato et al. 1984, Kallings et al. 1988), the Working Party on Immunizations (Beraadsgroep Immunisaties) of the National Health Council is still left with too many unanswered questions concerning effectiveness and safety to warrant switching to such a vaccine (Rümke 1988). Minor reactions following DPT/polio immunizations occur frequently. Local reactions, such as redness, swelling and pain occur following 30–50% of immunizations (Cody et al. 1981). The percentage rises to more than 80% when parents are asked about reactions (Swaak 1980). From approximately 2% of the immunizations upwards (1290 in total) reactions were a reason for consulting the general practitioner (Swaak 1980). When these figures are extrapolated from the total number of immunizations, we find that general practitioners are consulted approximately 20,000 times per year in connection with reactions following DPT/polio immunization. Reactions following immunizations against measles, or MMR immunizations as the case may be, are mostly unavoidable because these involve live, attenuated vaccine. There is no alternative available.

Both literally and figuratively, vaccines have a long way to go from production to injection. At numerous points along this route, unnecessary side effects can be produced by the wrong application of rules and regulations, for example, in transport and storage of vaccines, the wrong application of contraindications, and faulty injection techniques. The PEAs thoroughly inspect the 'cold chain' and the expiry dates. Vaccines are withdrawn whenever there is occasion to do so.

The contraindications are limited, but if they are not applied correctly this can either cause unnecessary morbidity or unnecessarily deprive children of immunizations (Rümke 1989b, Burgmeijer & Bolscher 1990, 1993). Unnecessary local reactions can also be caused by faulty injection techniques. The reorganization of the regional Community Health Care Organizations, which resulted in the falling away of the intermediate provincial structures, has made supervision of the proper implementation of the RVP more difficult. What effect this will have in the long term is still an open question.

2.2.1.3 Risks of immunization versus the risks of wild infection

Medical intervention (thus also immunization) can only be justified if the risks of the intervention are much smaller than the risks of abstinence. Table 3 lists the incidence of several complications, of undergoing the diseases (wild infection) compared with following immunization. The figures are to be taken as an indication because they can vary depending on the source (Cody et al. 1981, Barth 1984, White et al. 1985, Bol et al. 1987, Roosen & Van Aalderen 1989, Bol 1991). However, all sources report that the incidence of complications following a wild infection are much higher than after immunization.

Table 3 Incidence of serious complications in undergoing the disease, compared with immunizations

Complication		Infection	Incidence after immunization
D	death	1:20	0
P	convulsions	1:100	1:1750 to 1:2800
	brain damage	1:1000	< 1:400,000
	collapse		1:1750 to 1:2800
	death	1:100	0
T	death	1:2	0
Polio	paralysis	1:100 to 1:1000	0*
M	SSPE	1:100,000	0
	encephalitis	1:10,000	1:1,000,000
	pneumonia	1:100	0
	death	1:1000	0
R	CRS	1:14,000	0
Hib	meningitis	1:2400	0
	other major		
	Hib-diseases	1:2400	0

SSPE = Subacute sclerosing panencephalitis
CRS = Congenital rubella syndrome
* with Salk vaccine.

2.2.2 Effects at population level

2.2.2.1 Protection through herd immunity

The effectiveness of a series of immunizations is demonstrated on the one hand by a rise in the vaccine efficacy and, on the other hand, by a drop in the attack rate. The attack rate is the number of individuals who are ill, divided by the total number of individuals in the population. The attack rate drops within the group of non-immunized individuals as their ages rise, even though these individuals have not been immunized. This phenomenon can partly be explained by an increase in the number of individuals with natural immunity, but it can also be explained by herd immunity. When a high immunization uptake is achieved (90% or more), unprotected individuals within such a population are less likely to become infected.

They are, as it were, shielded by the mass of immunized individuals that surrounds them. In the case of a lower immunization uptake, the effect of herd immunity quickly disappears, and the pressure of infection will become relatively high and will considerably increase the chance of contracting the disease. In areas where many non-immunized individuals are concentrated, this can cause outbreaks of infectious diseases. The last three polio outbreaks in the Netherlands were in 1971, 1978 and 1992/1993 (Bijkerk et al. 1972, 1979, Huurman 1993). From the end of 1987 to the middle of 1988, an outbreak of measles was observed. Of the 1666 cases reported, 90% were non-immunized children. In 64% of these cases the parents' refusal of immunization were based on religious convictions, in 16% on an anthroposophical ideology (Bijkerk et al. 1989). The consequences for non-immune adults who travel abroad should not be disregarded: infection with measles or polio in adulthood has serious consequences.

2.2.2.2 Decreasing mortality and morbidity

The most effective weapon in the battle against infectious diseases is eradication of the source. This was achieved by a world-wide immunization programme against smallpox. The next most successful is blocking the route of infection, which is mostly achieved by general hygiene measures. However, the mediocre success of the public information campaigns against AIDS demonstrates that it is particularly difficult for human beings to block the route of infection through their behaviour as individuals. Specific raising of the resistance of the individual (immunization) only qualifies as third (Engel 1989).

Diphtheria (D)

A sharp drop in the incidence of diphtheria was observed in 1954. Two years earlier, the DPT vaccine had become available in the Netherlands and was being used on a large scale by the Child Health Clinics so that, by the time this immunization was introduced in the RVP in 1957, 70% of the children had already been immunized. Since the 1960s, there have never been more than three cases of diphtheria reported in any year, and in many years there were none at all. Practically speaking, diphtheria can be regarded as a disease that has disappeared in the Netherlands. But it can still be imported. Moreover, it must be remembered that immunized individuals may be carriers of *Corynebacterium diphtheriae* in the nasal cavity and on the skin. The fact that the disease no longer occurs does not mean that it no longer exists: therefore in the Netherlands too there is still a certain pressure of infection and there is no reason to change immunization policy.

Pertussis or whooping cough (P)

At the beginning of the 20th century, the infant mortality rate in the Netherlands was very high: more than 25% in some parts of the country. In addition to gastroenteritis and inadequate nutrition, diseases such as whooping cough and diphtheria contributed significantly to the high infant mortality rate (Meuleman 1906). As recently as 1946, whooping cough claimed 843 victims. Five years later the number of deaths had dropped to 128. Since large-scale immunizations were not introduced in the Netherlands until 1953, this drop must be attributed to improved conditions of social hygiene and to the larger-scale use of antibiotics in the treatment of complications. From 1965 onward, the mortality rate dropped practically to zero. In view of the alarming mortality and morbidity rates during the first half of this century, the side effects were negligible compared with the advantages of immunization. However, the weighing of advantages and disadvantages can have a different outcome when the mortality has fallen to zero and morbidity has become an exception. The whooping cough vaccine (and the P component in the DPT/polio vaccine) has remained essentially the same since it first became available (about 1930). Its side effects have likewise remained unchanged (Madsen 1933).

In the 1970s, particularly in the United Kingdom (Kulenkampff et al. 1974), Sweden and Germany, a battle was waged against the whooping cough immunization because of its (alleged) side effects. In Germany, in 1974, universal immunization against whooping cough was discouraged, and was limited to high-risk populations. In Sweden, the immunization was officially abolished in 1979. These matters were not without consequences: the immunization uptake in Britain dropped from approximately 75% in 1970 to 30% in 1978. In some areas it barely rose above 10%. In 1978, more than 65,000 cases of whooping cough were reported, 12 of which were fatal. Another gloomy peak was reached in 1982 with 14 dead. In Germany more than 80,000 cases were reported in 1980 (Hannik 1985), and in 1981 and 1982, 14 and 13 people died of whooping cough respectively (Pöhn 1984).

The reaction in the Netherlands was threefold, but less drastic. First, the concentration of *Bordetella pertussis* in the DPT/polio vaccine that had been used since 1962 was reduced from 16 opacity units (OU) to 10 OU in 1975. With 16 OU the vaccine was ample in relation to the international requirements of the WHO for the effectiveness of 4 IU (International Units). Even after reduction of the concentration of *B. pertussis*, the vaccine still met these WHO requirements. A second measure concerned the notification requirement for whooping cough in 1976. The third reaction, which followed in 1977, was to add to the official list of contraindications the occurrence of convulsions, not only in the child itself, but also in close relatives. In 1981, failure to observe this change led the Medical Disciplinary Tribunal (Medisch Tuchtcollege) to take measures against the doctor concerned (MTC 1981). Also in the Netherlands, an increasing number of cases of whooping cough were reported. There had only been 80 in 1982, but by 1986 the number had gone up to 2159. From various quarters a variety of explanations were given: a real increase in incidence, raised awareness in the medical profession, more frequent application of serodiagnostic procedures, increased pressure from abroad, and the reduction of concentration of the vaccine (Aronson et al. 1984, Bos 1984, Bijkerk 1984, Nagel et al. 1984, Nagelkerke 1984).

However, it appears that there was only a limited real increase in incidence, and that the explanation should primarily be sought in an increase in the use of serodiagnostic procedures and greater alertness of doctors. The reduced concentration of the vaccine did not have any influence, and there had probably never been any question of increased pressure of infection from abroad (Van der Water 1988). On the basis of these conclusions, a uniform definition of the disease was promulgated to ensure improved surveillance of whooping cough. In accordance with which reporting of cases was to take place from that moment on (Bijkerk 1988, Van der Water et al. 1988). As mentioned above in the discussion on side effects, a causal relationship between permanent neurological symptoms and whooping cough vaccine is no longer considered probable. In 1984, the concentration of the P component of the DPT/polio vaccine was brought back to 16 OU and in 1989, the contraindications were narrowed down again (Rümke 1989). In other countries there was also a retracing of steps: in Britain, immunization is being strongly propagated again (Sefi & Macfarlane 1989) and, in Germany the Ständige Impfkommission des Bundesgesundheitsamtes (Permanent Committee on Immunization of the Ministry of Health) quite recently included universal immunization against whooping cough in the German immunization schedule (Hartung 1991).

The effects of the recent measures in the Netherlands on the morbidity figures were predictable because, in order to diagnose whooping cough, two serum specimens need to be taken to determine the rise in titre of antibodies, and this definitely comes up against practical problems. It is, therefore, not surprising that the increase of the past years reversed into a sharp drop from 2709 notified cases in 1987 to 112 cases in 1988 (CBS 1991). Once again, the reported incidence of whooping cough in the Netherlands has become a rough estimate of the real situation. Nevertheless, as far as registration is concerned, the Netherlands compares favourably with its neighbours.

Tetanus (T)

A decreased incidence can also be observed in tetanus since the introduction of immunization (unofficially in 1952, officially in 1957), but because of the limited duration of the protection there has been a relative shift in its incidence from a younger age group to an older one. Considering the year in which this shift began, the effect must be attributed to immunization. But the decrease is definitely also the result of the adequate treatment of wounds in combination with the use of immunoglobulin. This passive protection lasts a few weeks. The number of cases of tetanus is quite small (< 5 per year). Neonatal tetanus is no longer seen. Because no immunity is built up as a result of a wild infection with *Clostridium tetani*, immunization will continue to be indispensable for protection.

Poliomyelitis (polio)

Polio is caused by a virus of which three forms are known: types 1, 2 and 3. Infection with one of the three does not result in immunity to the other types. For this reason, a trivalent vaccine is used in the Netherlands. The vaccine is of the Salk-type. Thanks to the RVP, the cases of polio are extremely low and limited to outbreaks that from time to time occur in certain subpopulations. Areas concerned are those where relatively many people live who refuse immunization on principle. The last three polio outbreaks were observed in 1971, 1978 and 1992/1993 (Bijkerk et al. 1972, 1979, Huurman 1993). In the event that a new outbreak of polio occurs or threatens, the Chief Medical Inspector recommends a number of measures to contain the danger. These measures should be made known in good time through channels intended for that purpose. However, an analysis of the last outbreak showed several major shortcomings in the measures taken. Firstly, a number of scientific questions that had been raised during the outbreak in 1978 had remained unanswered. Secondly, at the beginning of the outbreak there were two scenarios available and it was not clear which should be used. Thirdly, the communication between the Chief Medical Inspector and the District and Municipal Health Services (GGDs) was not efficient because of lack of organization and coordination on local and national levels (Huurman, 1993).

Haemophilus influenzae type b (Hib)

Infection with *Haemophilus influenzae type b*, particularly in children, can lead to serious complications including meningitis, epiglottitis and bacterial arthritis (Neijens et al. 1991). The incidence of meningitis caused by all bacterial pathogens together is estimated at 85–205 per 100,000 live births (Roord, 1989). Hib is one of these pathogens of bacterial meningitis with a relatively high occurrence particularly in the 0–4 year age group, with a peak at 8 months. Twelve per cent of the patients are younger than 5 months. Per year, approximately 700 children (mostly infants) will suffer a Hib infection (Bol 1991). Incidence rates in the Netherlands are based on the number of strains that have been sent to the Netherlands Reference Laboratory for Bacterial Meningitis (Nederlands Referentie Laboratorium voor Bacteriële Meningitis) since 1975, taking into account approximately 20% under-reporting (Spanjaard et al. 1985). In a retrospective study, a 2% lethality was found, and 8.7% of cases developed serious complications. A statistical relationship was found between the occurrence of otitis media and Hib meningitis. There is also a seasonal influence (higher during spring and autumn). The average and standard periods of hospitalization were 27 and 25 days, respectively (Bol et al. 1987) and are considerably longer than the usual periods in other countries (approximately 14 days).

Since 1 April 1993, the Hib immunization has been part of the RVP (Burgmeijer 1993). The immunization scheme is identical to the DPT/polio scheme (Table 1) and therefore the immunizations are administered by the staff of the Child Health Clinics. Within the RVP framework only the Pasteur-Mérieux conjugated PRP-T vaccine is used. The Hib immunizations in the RVP are given simultaneously with the DPT/polio immunizations (but as separate injections). So far, there are no signs of problems regarding the acceptance of the new immunization by the public. The development of a pentavalent DPT/polio/Hib vaccine is in progress, but since development of a new vaccine takes 5–10 years, a considerable time lag is to be expected.

Mumps (M)

Mumps is probably a generalized virus infection that, in the classical case, presents in the form of parotitis, but 20–40% of cases develop subclinically (Van der Veen 1979). Therefore, the notified cases of the disease are only a poor reflection of the real incidence of mumps. Most infections occur between the ages of 1 and 9 years. By the age of 15, 85% of children appear to have built up natural immunity. In 0.4% to 1.0% of cases, neurological complications develop (meningitis and encephalitis), more often in boys than in girls (2.5:1). Meningitis has a favourable prognosis, encephalitis may become more serious, but is seldom fatal. Before the introduction of the MMR immunization, two deaths per year were reported with mumps as the primary cause. Death from mumps is not a reason for universal immunization (De Jonge 1979). Orchitis occurs mainly after puberty, is usually unilateral, and consequently only very rarely results in sterility. In the Netherlands, an average of 400 patients per year are hospitalized with mumps. The average stay in hospital is 15 days. Absences from school due to mumps, per school day, is estimated at 1000. There are indications that the incidence of mumps has decreased since the introduction of the MMR immunization in 1987, but in connection with the irregular development of the incidence of mumps, and the negative effects of introducing mumps vaccine at a mature age, it has been recommended that the epidemiology of mumps be charted thoroughly after 1992 (end of the special MMR schedule for non-immunized children) (Bergink & Burger 1990). Its negative effects have been described, specifically in America, where mumps epidemics among adolescents and adults have been reported (Cochi et al. 1988a,b Kaplan et al. 1988).

Measles (M)

Measles as a cause of death showed a downward trend as early as 1976. But the effect of introducing immunization is unmistakable (Anonymous 1978a).

In infancy and early childhood, measles is in itself a fairly innocuous disease. Immunization therefore serves to prevent complications. In 5% to 15% of cases, secondary bacterial infections develop (otitis media, tracheobronchitis, bronchopneumonia). Encephalitis is seen in one to three patients out of 10,000. Because the disease is relatively rare (100–300 cases per year), it is not always recognized (Roosen & Van Aalderen 1989), or a false-positive diagnosis is made owing to confusion with other exanthematous infectious diseases. From the end of 1987 to the middle of 1988 there was an outbreak of measles, with the highest incidence in the provinces of Zeeland and Flevoland (44.5 and 42.6 cases per 100,000 inhabitants, respectively) (Bijkerk et al. 1989). Through the fast and adequate response of the Community Health Care in collaboration with the District Health Service DGD, the spread of the disease was kept within bounds (Burgmeijer 1988, DGD Flevoland 1989). From time to time local outbreaks of measles are reported, for example in Hilversum in 1992 (Fortuin 1993).

Rubella (R)

Rubella (German measles) is an acute viral infection that often develops with atypical symptoms or even subclinically. In itself, the disease does not constitute significant health (or health care) problems for either the individual or society. However, a primary infection in a pregnant woman can, even if the disease develops subclinically, result in serious deformities of the foetus. The risk of deformity depends on the stage of pregnancy and ranges from approximately 80% in the first month to about 10% in the fourth month. Such pregnancies often end in abortion or stillbirth. If a live child is born it may present a complex of symptoms known as the congenital rubella syndrome (CRS). CRS is characterized by deafness (87%), cardiovascular disorders (46%), mental retardation (39%), and cataract or glaucoma (34%). The death risk during the first year of life is 10% to 20% (Kuipers 1985).

Until 1974, approximately 100 children with CRS were born per year. Since 1974, all 11-year-old girls have had the opportunity of being immunized against rubella. Serological field studies carried out before the introduction of immunization showed that, by that age, 70% to 80% of girls had built up natural immunity (Houwert-de Jong et al. 1982, Van Druten et al. 1984a,b). Immunization, such as was carried out between 1974 and 1987, was intended to provide women with individual protection during their reproductive years. This strategy protected 98% to 99% of the target group. Despite the high percentage, approximately 50,000 women were still unprotected and each year a number of children were born with CRS. The numbers reported vary from 12 to 35 (Kuipers 1985, Van Wezel-Meijler et al. 1986). Because boys have also been immunized since the introduction of the MMR immunization in 1987, the circulation of the rubella virus will eventually come to a standstill. Simulation studies have shown that this will be the case after 5–10 years

(Knox 1980, Van Druten et al. 1984a,b, 1986). The incidence of CRS will decrease by 90%. The few individuals who are not immunized will then be protected by herd immunity.

There is another side to the new strategy: in relatively isolated communities, where immunization is refused, 90% of the women are still protected by natural immunity, because the virus keeps on circulating. When, as a result of the new strategy, this circulation comes to a standstill, the percentage of unprotected women in such communities could theoretically increase to 100%. In the event that the virus is imported into such a community, this could give rise to rubella epidemics and consequently also to an increase in the number of CRS cases. The chance of this happening is even greater because the birth rate in these communities is higher than the national average. Nevertheless, the total number of CRS cases in the Netherlands will decrease drastically with the new immunization strategy.

Hepatitis B (HB)

The HB immunization is not part of the RVP. On 1 October 1989, the screening of pregnant women for carriers of the hepatitis B surface antigen (HBsAg) was introduced at a national level. In the event of contact with the body fluid of a carrier, this antigen can cause hepatitis B. HBsAg can be demonstrated in most of the body fluids, such as blood, lymph, sperm, saliva, vomit, sputum, amniotic fluid, and breast milk. The first three are of particular importance. In cases of non-immunized children of HBsAg-positive mothers, it is recommended that the child should not be breast fed (Studiegroep Zuigelingenvoeding 1985). But this recommendation was dropped in the revised edition of the guidelines for infant feeding (GHI 1991b). Infection can occur vertically (from mother to newborn) or horizontally. In the case of the second route, sexual intercourse plays a very important role. The shared use of hypodermic needles by several people (drug addicts) is another route of infection that must not be disregarded. Therefore, in the Netherlands, most District and Municipal Health Services have a policy of making sterile needles and syringes easily available. Health workers can come into contact with contaminated blood accidentally, and thus become infected. In the non-surgical professions, however, the chance of this happening is extremely slight as long as normal measures of general hygiene are taken. Infection via transfusions with blood or blood products does not play a part in the Netherlands because these products are checked for HBsAg.

Linked to this screening is the immunization of children of mothers in whom HBsAg is found, which was also introduced nationwide on 1 October 1989. Because the timing of this immunization is linked to DPT/ polio immunizations (see Table 1), the implementation is largely carried out by the Child Health Clinics. Hence the discussion in this chapter. To support the nationwide introduction of hepatitis screening and immunization, the Medical Inspectorate published a bulletin (GHI 1989). Practical guidelines are available for the workers in the child health clinics (Burgmeijer & Bolscher 1990, 1993).

The average prevalence of HBsAg carriers among pregnant women is reported to lie between 0.8% and 0.9% (Mazel 1986, Martens 1989). This means that, with 200,000 pregnant women per year, there are between 1600 and 1800 carriers a year. In 29% of cases (which means 460 to 520 newborns) this results in perinatal HBV infection. The prognosis for these children is as follows: 20 children will develop acute ictero-hepatitis in the first year of life, one or two will die of fulminating hepatitis around the third month, more than 250 children will become HBsAg carriers and of these at least 90 will die of cirrhosis of the liver or of primary liver cell carcinoma between the 20th and 70th year of life. These figures seem small, but one should bear in mind that in the course of his/her life, each carrier will infect an average of 10 other people (Ypma et al. 1979). That is to say, the problem snowballs. Hepatitis B is a notifiable disease (group B). After a marked rise in the period 1969–1981, a decrease in the number of cases was observed which became more marked after 1985. This is probably the effect of changes in sexual behaviour, including protective measures taken in connection with AIDS. After 1990 however, the downward trend seems to have come to an end (Burgmeijer & Bolscher 1993).

The effect of the recently introduced screening and immunization programme is not as positive as had been expected at the time of introduction. The main reason for this seems to be that this immunization is not part of the RVP and thus cannot benefit from the good logistics and administration of the RVP (Grosheide & Klokman-Houweling 1993).

2.3 Costs of the RVP and the hepatitis B screening and immunization

2.3.1 Costs of the RVP

Recently, within the context of the 1992–1997 Long-Range Estimate of Home Care Services (Meerjarenraming Thuiszorg 1992–1997) an attempt was made to draw as complete a picture as possible of the costs of child health care from 0 to school age (Burgmeijer 1991). Table 4 lists the items that are associated with the implementation of the RVP.

Table 4 Costs involved in the implementation of the National
Immunization Programme of the Netherlands

Vaccines
  - production/purchase
  - storage
  - distribution
  - loss of vaccine
Administration
  - immunization records
  - office expenses
Materials
  - public information material
  - syringes, needles, disinfectants, swabs, adhesive tape
Staff
  - history taking (and physical examination) by the doctor
  - performance of the immunization by the doctor or the nurse
  - reimbursement of the Community Health Care services and GGDs
Support
  - PEA consultant community paediatrician
  - Medical Centre for Immunization of the RIVM
  - regular meetings between the Chief Medical Inspector and the PEA consultant
    community paediatricians
  - National Health Council Working Party on Immunizations (Beraadsgroep
    Immunisaties van de Gezondheidsraad)
  - training of staff

Costs generated by side effects

When this list is compared with most cost-effectiveness or cost-benefit
analyses in the literature, the incompleteness of the latter is immediately
obvious. This incompleteness was pointed out earlier (Cutting 1980).
Generally speaking, the costs in those analyses are limited to direct costs.
These are the costs associated with effectively carrying out the
immunizations. Sometimes they were even limited to a statement of the
production costs of the vaccines concerned. In 1990, the cost of vaccines
amounted to NLG 21.7 million (Annual report AWBZ 1991). Owing to the
recent introduction of the Hib immunization the cost of vaccines went up
to about 34 million. The implementing organizations are paid NLG 9.10
per immunization (total NLG 18.2 million), but in the case of the DPT/
polio and MMR vaccinations given at the child health clinics, this is settled
with the funds they receive from the AWBZ. The fact that immunizations
are being administered at about 2000 locations, means that an equivalent
number of refrigerators is needed to store the vaccine. On the basis of a cost
price of NLG 800 each, and a depreciation of 5 years, this generates an
annual cost of more than NLG 0.3 million. These costs are seldom included
in estimates. The item for the costs of the PEAs, about NLG 9 million, is
also rarely included in the estimate. The same applies to material costs

(approximately NLG 0.8 million) and the costs of carrying out the nearly 2 million injections per year (2,000,000 × 5 minutes × 60 cents per minute for the nurse's salary = 6 million guilders). In practice many injections are given by doctors, as a result of which the salary costs are approximately twice as high. Before the first immunization is administered (DPT/polio-1 + Hib-1 at 3 months), the doctor has to determine the indication on the basis of a case history and where necessary on the basis of the findings of a physical examination, which generates a cost item of approximately NLG 0.5 million. Without making detailed calculations, the item 'support and training' can definitely be estimated at NLG 1 million.

The total of the costs calculated above amounts to almost NLG 70 million per year. Because the sum of NLG 9 million for the PEAs includes the costs generated by the work of screening for PKU/CHT and the hepatitis B programme, the real direct costs of the RVP can, with some caution, be estimated at NLG 60–70 million per year. This does not include the indirect costs, costs that are for the greater part borne by the consumers. For example, travelling expenses, loss of wages, and costs that result from side effects. The 2% of cases in which the general practitioner is consulted in connection with immunization reactions alone lead to a cost of 0.6 million guilders.

2.3.2 Costs of hepatitis B screening and immunization

The costs generated by the PEAs are included in the 9 million that are listed under the costs of the RVP. The cost of blood sampling can be disregarded because the same blood sample also serves for blood group typing and testing for syphilis. Additional costs are generated by laboratory diagnosis and by administering immunizations to children of HBsAg-positive mothers. In 1990, the laboratory costs amounted to more than NLG 2.1 million (Annual report AWBZ 1991).

2.4 Cost-effectiveness and cost-benefit ratios

2.4.1 General

In determining cost-effectiveness ratios, more importance is attached to well-standardized methodology than to detailed itemization. This applies to the making of estimates on both the cost side and the effectiveness side (Van der Maas 1991). Models to determine standardized ratios in several divisions of the pre-school Child Health Care, have recently been developed under the direction of the Project on Integrated Evaluation of Child Health Care (Project Integrale Evaluatie Jeugdgezondheidszorg) and are being tested on the screening for hearing loss (De Koning et al. 1992).

2.4.2 National Immunization Programme (RVP)

Cost-effectiveness and cost-benefit analysis of the RVP are rare when it comes to DPT/polio and DT/polio immunizations. Analyses from other countries cannot be directly applied to the situation in the Netherlands because the immunization programmes and strategies differ. This applies particularly to analyses that concern developing countries. Both abroad and in the Netherlands, most analyses concern immunizations that were recently introduced: MMR, hepatitis B and Hib immunizations. In Switzerland, cost-benefit ratios of 1:2.0 and 1:1.2 were calculated for the separate measles and mumps immunizations, respectively, when only the direct costs were taken into consideration. When the indirect costs were also taken into account, the ratios became even more favourable, namely 1:5.0 and 1:2.6. The combined MMR immunization produced even better ratios of 1:2.9 (direct costs only) and 1:6.5 (direct costs plus indirect costs) (Just 1978, Barrazzoni et al. 1989). In the USA, the latter ratio was calculated at 1:14.0 (White et al. 1985). Although ratios mentioned in the literature vary, they are always positive.

2.4.3 Hepatitis B screening and immunization

Only analyses that concern the general introduction of screening plus immunization are discussed here. In other countries, the cost-benefit ratio of immunizations in certain select groups (for example, hospital staff) is currently under discussion. From these discussions it is clear that indirect costs are often not included, nor is the cost effectiveness of other aspects calculated in a standardized way, making it extremely difficult, if not impossible, to draw comparisons (Mulley et al. 1982, Botman et al. 1984, Heijtink & Schalm 1985a,b, Van der Ven et al. 1990).

In 1986, the Working Party on Hepatitis B Screening of Pregnant Women (Werkgroep Hepatitis B Screening voor Zwangeren) published a positive report on the introduction of screening and immunization. Among other things, this report was based on a positive cost-benefit analysis. The methodology used in this analysis was criticized for not making allowance for the so-called discount rate (applying the principle of interest). When a discount rate of 5% is calculated, the ratio swings to the negative side, and for each year of life gained, NLG 8,400 more costs are generated than if the immunization programme had not been carried out (Martens 1989). Nevertheless, the conclusion must be that screening plus immunization can be considered a relatively cost-effective provision. A discussion has started about the functionality of the laboratory aspect in particular (Rechsteiner 1990, Verbrugge 1990b). The importance of this and other points of discussion was tested in an evaluation study, which showed several weak points in the hepatitis B programme of the Netherlands (Grosheide & Klokman-Houweling 1993).

2.4.4 Haemophilus influenzae type B immunization

In anticipation of the introduction of the Hib immunization on 1 April 1993, cost-effectiveness ratios had been calculated in which allowance had been made for various cost factors. It was demonstrated that particularly the price of the vaccine greatly influences the ratio. On the basis of three immunizations at NLG 17.50 each, the costs of the immunization programme are not more than NLG 11,000 for each year of life gained. With a price rise or drop of 10%, this amount is increased or decreased, respectively, by 80% (Martens et al. 1991). In the case of a series of three immunizations and a vaccine price of NLG 15 or less, the balance swings to the positive side; with a price between NLG 15 and 20, the costs rise to a maximum of NLG 25,000 per year of life gained. The price of the vaccine used in the RVP is about NLG 15 per immunization, but the complete series consists of four instead of three, so the costs per year of life gained can be expected to be higher than NLG 25,000. This amount compares favourably with other health care provisions (Martens et al. 1991). Other factors that have a relatively strong influence on the cost-effectiveness ratio are the degree of protection provided by the vaccine, and the incidence of Hib meningitis.

2.5 Conclusions

On the basis of the available literature it can be said that the present immunizations in the Netherlands are highly effective. The effectiveness is demonstrated by the fact that, after the introduction of immunizations against diphtheria, whooping cough, tetanus, polio, measles and rubella, the incidence rates went down to the present, extremely low, levels. Even though, as a result of improvements in conditions of social hygiene and the availability of sophisticated diagnostic procedures and therapeutics, the drop in mortality and morbidity rates had already started before immunization was introduced. The effect of the introduction of each immunization is clearly demonstrable.

The immunizations of the RVP have a relatively positive cost-benefit ratio, that is to say that the RVP produces a large gain in health for the whole population for relatively low costs. The negative effects of the immunizations given in the Netherlands can be disregarded at population level and the risks for the individual are so low as to be acceptable. The monitoring and evaluation of side effects of immunizations is well organized. The discouraging of immunizations, other than on the grounds of the very limited contraindications, must be considered an unprofessional attitude by the doctor involved.

More and better simulation and evaluation studies are available for the immunizations that were introduced recently (MMR, HB and Hib) than for the immunizations that have been given for a long time.

Considering the wide range of the RVP, Child Health Clinics obviously offer a good infrastructure for implementing the National Immunization Programme.

The low incidence of infectious diseases against which the RVP offers protection justifies neither changing the immunization strategy, nor settling for a lower immunization uptake.

2.6 Recommendations

- It is recommended that the RVP with its executive, administrative, monitoring and evaluation functions be maintained. In connection with the reorganization of the Community Health Care Organizations and the PEAs, and the PEAs switch to a new computerized administration system on 1 January 1993, alertness is required to ensure that these functions are maintained.
- It is recommended that an evaluation study is always carried out some time after the introduction of a new immunization. The simulation studies and cost-effectiveness or cost-benefit analyses made beforehand should also be assessed.
- When introducing new immunizations, a small change in the price of a vaccine proves to have great impact on the outcome of the cost-benefit analysis. It is recommended that this be taken into account in the choice between several vaccines of equal quality.
- Children who qualify for both the RVP immunizations and the HB and BCG immunization are now receiving 14 injections during the first 14 months of their lives. Most of these should be given simultaneously, that is to say three or four injections at the same time. It is feared that in these

cases acceptance will be reduced and drop out from the programme may be the result. Yet not immunizing simultaneously pushes up costs. For these reasons it is recommended that new combined vaccines be developed to allow a reduction in the number of injections.

References

ACIP (Advisory Committee on Immunization Practices): Diphtheria, Tetanus, and Pertussis: Recommendations for Vaccine Use and Other Preventive Measures Centers for Disease Control, *Morbidity & Mortality Weekly Report* 40 (1991) No.RR-10.

Anonymous: Sterfte door mazelen en kinkhoest, *Info Bulletin JGZ* 10 (1978) 21.

Aronson D.C., Pilon, J.W., Blij, J.F. van der: Pertussispreventie; een kink in de kabel?, *Nederlands Tijdschrift voor Geneeskunde* 128 (1984) 1412–1415.

Avery, M.E., First, A.L., Huang, A.: Infectious diseases, in: Avery, M.E. & First, L.R.: *Pediatric Medicine*, Baltimore: Williams & Wilkins, 1989.

AWBZ (Stichting Centraal Administratiekantoor AWBZ): *Jaarverslag over 1990*, Den Haag 1991.

Ball, A.P. & Gray, J.A.: *Infectious diseases*, Edinburgh: Churchill Livingstone, 1984.

Barazzoni, F., Bourguin, M., Haber, J. et al. (Fachgruppe für Impffragen): *Eliminiation von Masern, Mumps und Röteln in der Schweiz*, Revidierte Auflage RECOM, Bern 1989.

Barth, P.G.: Kinkhoestvaccinatie bij kinderen met een neurologische afwijking, *Nederlands Tijdschrift voor Geneeskunde* 128 (1984) 1423–1424.

Bergink, A.H. & Burger, I.: Bof in Den Haag in 1984, *Tijdschrift voor Jeugdgezondheidszorg* 22 (1990) 58–60.

Bijkerk, H.: Neemt kinkhoest werkelijk toe?, *Nederlands Tijdschrift voor Geneeskunde* 128 (1984) 1421–1422.

Bijkerk, H.: Het nut van de immunisatie tegen kinkhoest, *Nederlands Tijdschrift voor Geneeskunde* 130 (1986) 41–42 (a).

Bijkerk, H.: *Rationalization of immunization schedules*, Paper presented for the European Advisory Group on EPI WHO, Copenhagen 1986 (b).

Bijkerk, H., Draaisma, F.J., Landheer, T., et al.: Poliomyelitis in Staphorst, *Nederlands Tijdschrift voor Geneeskunde* 116 (1972) 549–558.

Bijkerk, H., Draaisma, F.J., Gugten, A.G. et al.: De poliomyelitis-epidemie in 1978, *Nederlands Tijdschrift voor Geneeskunde* 123 (1979) 1700–1714.

Bijkerk, H., Bilkert-Mooiman, M.A.J., Houtters, H.J.: De inentingstoestand bij aangegeven patiënten met mazelen tijdens de epidemie 1987/'88, *Nederlands Tijdschrift voor Geneeskunde* 133 (1989) 29–32.

Bol, P.: Epidemiologie van Haemophilus influenzae type-b infecties in Nederland en elders, *Nederlands Tijdschrift voor Geneeskunde* 135 (1991) 7–9.

Bol, P., Spanjaard, L., Arends, A., Zanen, H.C.: Epidemiology of Haemophilus influenzae meningitis in children 0–6 years of age, in: Bol, P.: *Epidemiology of bacterial meningitis in The Netherlands*, Amsterdam 1987 (dissertatie).

Boo, T.M. de, Druten, J.A.M. van, Lemmens, W.A.J.G. et al.: Rubella: dynamische effecten na wijziging van het vaccinatieprogramma, *Tijdschrift voor Sociale Gezondheidszorg* 64 (1986) 822–829.

Bos, S.E.: Kinkhoest, *Nederlands Tijdschrift voor Geneeskunde* 128 (1984) 1409–1411.

Botman, M.J., Botterhuis, J.A.M., Krieger, R.A.: Immunisatie tegen hepatitis B; kosten en baten in een Nederlands ziekenhuis, *Nederlands Tijdschrift voor Geneeskunde* 128 (1984) 1748–1752.

Burgmeijer, R.J.F.: *Circulaire voor de CB-teams d.d. 28 januari 1988*, Dronten: Stichting Kruiswerk Provincie Flevoland, 1988.

Burgmeijer, R.J.F.: *Kostenraming JGZ*, Bunnik: LVT, 1991 (interne notitie).

Burgmeijer, R.J.F.: Uitbreiding van het Rijksvaccinatieprogramma met Hib-vaccinatie. *MGZ* (1993) 21(3) 17–21.

Burgmeijer, R.J.F. & Bolscher, D.J.A.: *Richtlijnen voor de uitvoering van het Rijksvaccinatieprogramma*, Zwolle: Entadministratie voor de provincies Overijssel en Flevoland, 1990.

Burgmeijer, R.J.F. & Bolscher, D.J.A.: *Vaccinaties bij Kinderen; uitvoering en achtergronden van het Rijksvaccinatieprogramma en andere vaccinaties bij kinderen*. Assen: Van Gorcum publishers, 1993.

CBS (Centraal Bureau voor de Statistiek): *Statistisch jaarboek 1991*, Den Haag: Sdu Uitgeverij, 1991.

Cochi, S.L., Preblud, S.R., Orenstein, W.A.: Perspectives on the relative resugence of mumps in the United States I, *American Journal of Diseases of Children* 142 (1988) 499–507 (a).

Cochi, S.L., Preblud, S.R., Orenstein, W.A.: Perspectives on the relative resugence of mumps in the United States II, *American Journal of Diseases of Children* 142 (1988) 1021–1022 (b).

Cody, C.L., Baraff, L.J., Cherry, J.D. et al.: The nature and rate of adverse reactions associated with DTP and DT immunization in infants and children, *Pediatrics* 68 (1981) 650–660.

Cutting, W.A.M.: Cost-benefit evaluations of vaccination programmmes, *Lancet* (1980) 634–635.

DGD (Districtsgezondheidsdienst) Flevoland: *Jaarverslag 1988*, Lelystad: DGD Flevoland, 1989.

Druten, J.A.M. van, Boo, T. de, Doesburg, W.H. et al.: Incidentie van het congenitale rubellasyndroom; een mathematisch-epidemiologische benadering; enkele implicaties voor de epidemiologie van rubella en het vaccinatiebeleid in Nederland, *Tijdschrift voor Sociale Gezondheidszorg* 62 (1984) 438–446 (a).

Druten, J.A.M. van, Boo, T. de, Reintjes, A.G.M.: *Rubella-vaccinatie; effecten op lange termijn van alternatieve strategieën, Rapport bestemd voor de Commissie Bof- en Rubellavaccinatie van de Gezondheidsraad*, Nijmegen/Bilthoven 1984 (b).

Druten, J.A.M. van, Boo, T. de, Doesburg, W.H. et al.: Rubellavaccinatie; effecten op lange termijn van alternatieve strategieën, *Tijdschrift voor Sociale Gezondheidszorg* 64 (1986) 210–218.

Engel, H.W.B.: Preventie van infectieziekten en meting van de doeltreffendheid daarvan; Infectieziektenbewaking, een permanente noodzaak, *Nederlands Tijdschrift voor Geneeskunde* 133 (1989) 861–862.

Fortuin, H.B. Mazelen-epidemie zomer 1992. *Infectieziektenbulletin* 1993 (4), 2–8.

Gezondheidsraad: *Encephalitis postvaccinalis en andere verwikkelingen ten gevol- ge van vaccinatie*, Den Haag: Staatsuitgeverij, 1972.

Gezondheidsraad: *Ongewenste bijwerkingen vaccins Rijksvaccinatie-program- ma in 1985*, Den Haag 1986.

Gezondheidsraad: *Ongewenste bijwerkingen vaccins Rijksvaccinatie-program- ma in 1986*, Den Haag 1987.

Gezondheidsraad: *Ongewenste bijwerkingen vaccins Rijksvaccinatie-program- ma in 1987*, Den Haag 1988.

Gezondheidsraad: *Ongewenste bijwerkigen vaccins Rijksvaccinatie-program- ma in 1988*, Den Haag 1989.

Gezondheidsraad: *Bijwerkingen vaccins Rijksvaccinatieprogramma in 1990*, Den Haag 1991.

GHI: *Vaccinatietoestand Nederland per 1 september 1980*, Leidschendam 1981 (a).

GHI: *GHI Bulletin: Praktische wenken inzake (re)vaccinaties in het kader van het Rijksinentingsprogramma*, Leidschendam 1981 (b).

GHI: *GHI Bulletin: Preventie Hepatitis B bij pasgeborenen*, Rijswijk 1989.

GHI: *Vaccinatietoestand Nederland per 1 januari 1990*, Rijswijk 1991 (a).

GHI: *GHI Bulletin: Zuigelingenvoeding; Uitgangspunten en praktische aanbeve-lingen*, Rijswijk 1991 (b).

GHI: *Vaccinatietoestand Nederland per 1 januari 1991*, Rijswijk 1992.

Grosheide, P.M. & Klokman-Honweling, J.M.: Hepatitis B-vaccinatie van neonaten geboren in 1990. Bilthoven: *RIVM*, 1993.

Hannik, C.A.: *Verslag van de Geneeskundige Hoofdinspecteur over de Vaccinatie-campagne tegen poliomyelitis gedurende de jaren 1957–1962*, Den Haag: Staats-uitgeverij, 1963.

Hannik, C.A.: Kinkhoest, in: Huisman, J. (red.): *Immunisatie tegen infectie-ziekten*, Alphen a/d Rijn: Stafleu, 1984.

Hannik, C.A.: Vaccinatie tegen kinkhoest, *Tijdschrift voor Therapie, Geneesmiddel en Onderzoek* 10 (1985) 695–697.

Hartung, K.: Die neuen Impfempfehlungen der Ständigen Impfkommission des Bundesgesundheitsamtes, *Sozialpädiatrie* 13 (1991) 559–560.

Heijtink, R.A. & Schalm, S.W.: Hepatitis B vaccinatie bij neonaten van HBsAg positieve moeders, *Tijdschrift voor Therapie, Geneesmiddel en Onderzoek* 10 (1985) 698–701 (a).

Heijtink, R.A. & Schalm, S.W.: Hepatitis B-immunisatie in Nederlandse ziekenhuizen, *Nederlands Tijdschrift voor Geneeskunde* 129 (1985) 291–294 (b).

Houwert-de Jong, M.H., Lindert, A.C.M. van, Alsbach, G.P.J. et al.: Besmetting met rubellavirus tijdens de zwangerschap, *Nederlands Tijdschrift voor Geneeskunde* 126 (1982) 1738–1739.

Huisman, J.: De immunisatie tegen infectieziekten; enkele recente aspecten van de 'vaccinologie', *The Practitioner* (1985) 809–816.

Huurman, J.G.J. *Bestrijding polio-epidemie 1992–1993; procesevaluatie in opdracht van het ministerie van WVC.* Wassenaar: Huurman Consult b.v., 1993.

Jefferson, N., Sleight, G., Macfarlane, A.: Immunization of children by a nurse without a doctor present, *British Medical Journal* 294 (1987) 423–424.

Jonge, G.A. de: Bofmeningitis en bofsterfte, *Tijdschrift voor Jeugdgezondheidszorg* 11 (1979) 91–93.

Just, M.: Rentiert die Masern- und/oder Mumps-Impfung für Schweizerische Verhältnisse?, *Schweizerisches Medizinisches Wochenschrift* 108 (1978) 1763–1768.

Kallings, L.O., Olin, P., Storsater, J.: Placebo-controlled trial of two avellular pertussis vaccines in Sweden; Protective efficacy and adverse events, *Lancet* (1988) 955–960.

Kaplan, K.M., Marder, D.C., Cochi, S.L. et al.: Mumps in the Workplace; Further evidence of the changing epidemiology of a childhood vaccine-preventable disease, *Journal of The American Medical Association* 260 (1988) 1434–1438.

Knox, E.G.: Strategy for Rubella Vaccination, *International Journal of Epidemiology* 9 (1980) 13–23.

Koning, H.J. de, Juttman, R.E. of Panman, J. *Kosten–effectiviteitsanalyse in de jengdgezondheidszorg voor 0–4 jarigen: methoden en mogelijkheden*, *Rotterdam:* Instituut voor Maatschappelijke Gezondheidszorg, 1993.

Kuipers, F.: Het voorkomen van congenitale rubella, *Nederlands Tijdschrift voor Geneeskunde* 129 (1985) 211–2114.

Kulenkampff, M., Schwarzman, J.S., Wilson, J.: Neurological Complications of Pertussis Inoculation, *Archives of Disease in Childhood* 49 (1974) 46–49.

LVT (Landelijke Vereniging voor Thuiszorg): *Nota Medisch Handelen door Verpleegkundig Beroepsbeoefenaren in de Thuissituatie*, Deel 1 2^e druk, Deel 2 2^e herziene druk, Bunnik: LVT, 1991.

Maas, P.J. van der: Kosten-effectiviteitsvraagstellingen in de jeugdgezondheidszorg, *Tijdschrift voor Jeugdgezondheidszorg* 23 (1991) 45–46.

Madsen, T.: Vaccination against whooping cough, *Journal of the American Medical Association* 101 (1933) 187–188.

Martens, L.L.: De kosten-effectiviteit van screening van zwangeren op hepatitis B, *Tijdschrift voor Sociale Gezondheidszorg* 67 (1989) 379–381.

Martens, L.L., Velden, G.H.M. ten, Bol, P.: De kosten en baten van vaccinatie tegen Haemophilus influenzae type b, *Nederlands Tijdschrift voor Geneeskunde* 135 (1991) 16–20.

Mazel, J.A.: *Preventie van perinatale Hepatitis B bij pasgeborenen in Nederland*, Rotterdam 1986 (dissertatie).

Meuleman, C.: *Het levensrecht van de geboren vrucht*, Bussum: Paul Brand, 1906.

Miller, D., Ross, E.M., Alderslade, R. et al.: Pertussis immunization and serious acute neurological illness in children, *British Medical Journal* 282 (1981) 1595–1599.

Ministerie van Volksgezondheid en Milieuhygiëne: *Besluit Uitvoering Vaccinatie- programma Bijzondere Ziektekostenverzekering*, Leidschendam 26 juni 1974 (a).

Ministerie van Volksgezondheid en Milieuhygiëne: *Besluit Verstrekken van Inlichtingen door de Gemeentebesturen aan de Provinciale Entadministraties*, Leidschendam 19 augustus 1974 (b).

Ministerie van Volksgezondheid en Milieuhygiëne: *Besluit van 16 mei 1974 houdende wijziging van het Verstrekkingenbesluit Bijzondere Ziektekosten-verzekering 1968*, Leidschendam 16 mei 1974 (c).

Ministerie van Volksgezondheid en Milieuhygiëne: *Besluit tot Opnememing van Mazelenvaccinatie t.b.v. vier- en negenjarige kinderen in het vaccinatieprogramma*, Leidschendam 27 mei 1977.

Ministerie van Volksgezondheid en Milieuhygiëne: *Besluit Erkenningsnormen Kruisorganisaties*, Leidschendam 1 juni 1981.

MTC (Medisch Tuchtcollege 's-Gravenhage): Uitspraak inzake klacht DKTP in plaats van DTP-vaccin, *Medisch Contact* (1981) 1513.

Mulley, A.G., Silverstein, M.D., Dienstag, J.L.: Indications for use of hepatitis B vaccine, based om cost-effectiveness analysis, *New England Journal of Medicine* 307 (1982) 644–651.

Nagel, J., Graaf, S. de, Schijf-Evers, D.: Serodiagnose van kinkhoest, *Nederlands Tijdschrift voor Geneeskunde* 129 (1984) 1427–1428.

Nagelkerke, A.F.: Steekt kinkhoest de kop weer op?, *Tijdschrift voor Jeugdgezondheidszorg* 16 (1984) 40–42.

Neijens, H.J., Groot, R. de, Dzoljic-Danilovic, G.: Haemophilus influenzae type b-infecties bij kinderen, *Nederlands Tijdschrift voor Geneeskunde* 135 (1991) 13–16.

Pöhn, H.P.: Gesundheitsgefährdung unserer Kinder durch Infektionskrankheiten, *Bundesgesundheitsblatt* 27 (1984) 118–121.

Rechsteiner, J.: De preventie van hepatitis B bij pasgeborenen kan doelmatiger worden georganiseerd, *Medisch Contact* 45 (1990) 549.

Roord, J.J.: Richtlijnen bacteriële meningitis bij kinderen, *Nederlands Tijdschrift voor Geneeskunde* 133 (1989) 831–834.

Roosen, Y.M. & Aalderen, W.M.C. van: Mazelen, ook in deze tijd nog een probleem?, *Nederlands Tijdschrift voor Geneeskunde* 133 (1989) 1009–1011.

Ruitenberg, E.J.: Vaccinologie: het ontwikkelen, bereiden, controleren en toe passen van vaccins, *Nederlands Tijdschrift voor Geneeskunde* 133 (1989) 863–864.
Ruitenberg, E.J., Bos, J.M., Elgersma, A.: Vaccinatie, *Tijdschrift voor Sociale Gezondheidszorg* 62 (1984) 205–210.

Rümke, H.C.: Een beter vaccin tegen kinkhoest?, *Nederlands Tijdschrift voor Geneeskunde* 132 (1988) 2192–2194.

Rümke, H.C.: Contra-indicaties tegen vaccinaties in het Rijksvaccinatie-programma, *Nederlands Tijdschrift voor Geneeskunde* 133 (1989) 1975–1977.

Sato, Y., Kimura, M., Fukumi, H.: Development of a pertussis component vaccine in Japan, *Lancet* (1984) 122–126.

Sefi, S. & Macfarlane, A.: *Immunizing children*, Oxford: Oxford Medical Publications, 1989.

Spanjaard, L., Bol, P., Ekker, W. et al.: De incidentie van bacteriële meningitis in Nederland; vergelijking van drie registratiesystemen, *Nederlands Tijdschrift voor Geneeskunde* 129 (1985) 355–359.

Stel, A. van der: Kinderziektes; Inenten: Ja of nee? *Jonas* (1986) 10–12.

Stoop, J.W. & Vossen, J.M.J.J.: Infectieziekten, in: Brande, J.L. van den, Gelderen, H.H. van, Monnens, L.A.H. (red.): *Kindergeneeskunde*, Utrecht: Wetenschappelijke Uitgeverij Bunge, 1990.

Studiegroep Zuigelingenvoeding: *Zuigelingenvoeding; Algemene uitgangspunten en praktische aanbevelingen*, Bunnik/Den Haag: Nationale Kruisvereniging/Voorlichtingsbureau voor de Voeding, 1985.

Swaak, A.J.: Reacties op DKTP-vaccin, *Medisch Contact* (1980) 1061–1064.

Veen, J. van der: Algemene enting tegen bof?, *Nederlands Tijdschrift voor Geneeskunde* 123 (1979) 714–715.

Ven, A.A.H. van de, Hattum, J. van, Willers, J.M.N.: De kosten van hepatitis B-vaccinatie: een herbeschouwing, *Nederlands Tijdschrift voor Geneeskunde* 134 (1990) 298–301.

Verbrugge, H.P.: Vaccinatie van prematuur geboren kinderen, *Nederlands Tijdschrift voor Geneeskunde* 130 (1986) 42.

Verbrugge, H.P.: Een irreële veronderstelling (antwoord op Rechsteiner 1990), *Medisch Contact* 45 (1990) 549.

Water, H.P.A. van de: Kinkhoestaangiften in Nederland in de periode 1976–1986 en de noodzaak van een uniforme ziektedefinitie, *Nederlands Tijdschrift voor Geneeskunde* 132 (1988) 821–828.

Water, H.P.A. van de, Laar, M.J.W. van de, Leentvaar-Kuipers, A.: Wanneer is het kinkhoest? Verband tussen laboratoriumdiagnostische bevindingen en klachten, *Nederlands Tijdschrift voor Geneeskunde* 132 (1988) 828–833.

Wezel-Meijler, G. van, Gerards, L.J., Fleer, A., et al.: Het congenitale rubellasyndroom; een nog niet verdwenen ziektebeeld, *Nederlands Tijdschrift voor Geneeskunde* 130 (1986) 1793–1796.

White, C.C., Koplan, J.P., Orenstein, W.A.: Benefits, risks and costs of immunization for measles, mumps and rubella, *American Journal of Public Health* 75 (1985) 739–744.

Ypma, T.D., Kater, L., Gerards, L.J. et al.: Perinataal verworven virushepatitis B, *Nederlands Tijdschrift voor Geneeskunde* 123 (1979) 1820–1828.

Further reading

Anonymous: Kinkhoestvaccinatie, *Info Bulletin JGZ* 10 (1978) 49–51.

Ament, A.J.H.A., Sprenger, M., Botman, M.J. et al.: Kostenbatenanalyse van vaccinatie tegen pneumococcenpneumonie, *Nederlands Tijdschrift voor Geneeskunde* 130 (1986) 407–410.

Bijkerk, H.: Het nationale vaccinatieprogramma; nu en in de toekomst, *Tijdschrift voor Therapie, Geneesmiddel en Onderzoek* 10 (1985) 663–668.

Bijkerk, H.: Informatie kinkhoestaangifte, *Nederlands Tijdschrift voor Geneeskunde* 132 (1988) 833–834.

Brands-Bottema, G.W.: Overheidsdwang bij vaccinatie?, *Nederlands Juristenblad* 39 (1988) 1412–1414.

Bulsink, C. & Gosselink, I: *De organisatie van en voorlichting over inentingen, in het bijzonder bij negenjarigen*, Wageningen: Landbouwuniversiteit Wageningen, 1988 (doctoraalscriptie Gezondheidsleer).

Burgmeijer, R.J.F. & Bolscher, D.J.A.: *Richtlijnen voor de uitvoering van de Hepatitis-B-vaccinatie bij zuigelingen van HBsAg-positieve moeders*, Zwolle: Entadministratie voor de provincies Overijssel en Flevoland, 1990.

Coutinho, R.A.: Virale hepatitis, *Tijdschrift voor Sociale Gezondheidszorg* 62 (1984) 228–232.

Drewes, J.B.J.: Belangrijke wijziging vaccinatieprogramma, *Maatschappelijke Gezondheidszorg* 14 (1986) 12–14.

Geelen, S.P.M.: *Bacteriële meningitis; klinische en epidemiologische gegevens*, Lezing Wilhelmina Kinderziekenhuis, Utrecht 22-4-1991.

Gezondheidsraad: *Rapport rodehond-vaccin*, Den Haag: Staatsuitgeverij, 1971.

Gezondheidsraad: *Advies inzake het invoeren van een vaccinatieplicht en het effect daarvan op de inentingsgraad van de bevolking*, Den Haag: Staatsuitgeverij, 1975.

Gezondheidsraad: *Advies inzake Anti-HBs in transfusiebloed en Anti-Hepatitis B Immunoglobuline concentraten bij de prophylaxe van Hepatitis B*, Den Haag: Staatsuitgeverij, 1979.

Gezondheidsraad: *Advies inzake pneumococcen immunisatie*, Den Haag: Staatsuitgeverij, 1982 (a).

Gezondheidsraad: *Advies inzake poliomyelitis*, Den Haag: Staatsuitgeverij, 1982 (b).

Gezondheidsraad: *Advies inzake Bof-/rubellavaccinatie*, Den Haag: Staatsuit-geve-rij, 1984.

Gezondheidsraad: *Bijwerkingen vaccins Rijksvaccinatieprogramma in 1989*, Den Haag 1990.

GHI (Geneeskundige Hoofdinspectie van de Volksgezondheid): *Nota betreffende de Uitvoering van het Vaccinatieprogramma*, Leidschendam 1979.

GHI: *GHI Bulletin: Borstvoeding*, Rijswijk 1987.

GHI: *GHI Bulletin: De aangifte van infectieziekten*, Rijswijk 1988.

Goulet, V. & Papasoglou, S.: Evaluation de la couverture vaccinale "rougeole" et "rubeole" sur le plan national a partir d'un echantillon d'écoles, *Annales de Pediatrie* (Paris) 36 (1989) 43–48.

Grosheide, P.M.: Hepatitis B vaccinatie, hoe vaker hoe beter?, *SOA-Bulletin* 11 (1990) 3–4.

Gudnadottir, M.: Cost-effectiveness of different strategies for prevention of congenital rubella infection: a practical example from Iceland, *Reviews of Infectious Diseases* 7 Suppl 1 (1985) 200–209.

Gunning-Schepers, L.: Kleuterbureaus voor multiculturele groepen in Amsterdam; deelname aan het vaccinatie en gehoorscreeningsprogramma door Nederlandse en buitenlandse kinderen, *Tijdschrift voor Sociale Geneeskunde* 59 (1981) 471–477.

Hall, D.M.B., Hill, P., Elliman, D.: *The Child Surveillance Handbook*, Oxford: Radcliffe Medical Press, 1990.

Hinman, A.R.: Immunizations in the United States, *Pediatrics* 86 Suppl (1990) 1064–1066.

Hinman, A.R. & Koplan, J.P.: Pertussis and pertussis vaccine; reanalysis of benefits, risks, and costs, *Journal of the American Medical Association*, 251 (1984) 3109–3113.

Hinman, A.R., Bart, K.J., Hopkins, D.R.: Costs of not eradicating measles, *American Journal of Public Health* 75 (1985) 713–714.

Huber, E.G.: Pertussis und Pertussis-Impfstoffe, *Sozialpädiatrie* 13 (1991) 547–550.

Huisman, J. (red.): *Immunisatie tegen infectieziekten*, Alphen a/d Rijn: Stafleu, 1984.

Huisman, J.: Bijwerkingen van het Rijksvaccinatieprogramma in 1986, *Nederlands Tijdschrift voor Geneeskunde* 132 (1988) 5–6.

Johannesson, M., Jönsson, B.: Economic evaluation in health care: Is there a role for cost-benefit analysis? *Health Policy*, 17 (1991) 1–23.

Jonge, G.A. de: DTP of DKTP?, *Tijdschrift voor Jeugdgezondheidszorg* 14 (1982) 10–11.

Kamerbeek, A.E.H.M.: De Rubella-Werkgroep 21 juni 1947–1 januari 1983, *Medisch Contact* (1983) 479–480.

Kapsenberg, J.G.: De jacht op het poliovirus is geopend, *Nederlands Tijdschrift voor Geneeskunde* 133 (1989) 864–866.

Kock, M. de & Moorrees, M.: *Informatiebronnen welke een rol spelen bij de DKTP- en BMR-vaccinatie bij ouders met kinderen van 14 maanden*, Wageningen: Landbouwuniversiteit Wageningen, 1990 (doctoraalscriptie Gezondheidsleer).

Kuiper, C.M., Schlesinger-Was, E.A., Vaandrager, G.J.: Preventieve gezondheidszorg voor kinderen van migranten; een onderzoek naar de deelname aan de jeugdgezondheidszorg (0–4 jr) in Den Haag, *Tijdschrift voor Sociale Gezondheidszorg* 64 (1986) 365–369.

Laar, M.J.W. van de, Water, H.P.A. van de, Leentvaar-Kuipers, A.: Surveillance van kinkhoest in Amsterdam via aangiften uit peilstationpraktijken, *Nederlands Tijdschrift voor Geneeskunde* 132 (1988) 819–821.

Lafarge, H., Levy, E., Rey, M.: L'évaluation des politiques de vaccination; le cas de la rougéole, *Revue d'Epidemiologie et de Santé Publique* 33 (1985) 182–193.

Lim-Feyen, J.F.: *De buitenlandse zuigeling en de GG & GD Jeugdgezondheidszorg te Amsterdam*, Leiden: NIPG/TNO, 1983 (scriptie opleiding Jeugdgezondheidszorg).

Lozekoot, J., Teunissen-De Zeeuw, M., Vries-Lequin, I. de: *Een onderzoek naar de vaccinatiegraad van kinderen van migranten*, Tiel: Gemeenschappelijke Gezondheidsdienst Rivierenland, 1990.

Mazel, J.A. & Schalm, S.W.: Screening van zwangeren; Waarom zwangere vrouwen systematisch moeten worden onderzocht op HBsAg, *Medisch Contact* 40 (1985) 776–780.

Mazel, J.A., Heijtink, R.A., Schalm, S.W. et al.: Gecombineerde passieve en actieve immunisatie van zuigelingen van HBsAg-positieve moeders, *Nederlands Tijdschrift voor Geneeskunde* 129 (1985) 590–594.

Medicine Group, The: *Highlights of an international workshop on Haemophilus influenzae type b: The role of vaccination*, Oxford 1989.

Mulder, C.J.J.: Neonatale meningitis in Nederland 1976–1977, *Nederlands Tijdschrijft voor Geneeskunde* 123 (1979) 1832–1836.

Mulder, C.J.J.: *Neonatal meningitis in The Netherlands*, Amsterdam 1984 (dissertatie).

Mulder, C.J.J.: Etiologie en epidemiologie van neonatale meningitis, *The Practitioner* (1985) 771–774.

NK (Nationale Kruisvereniging): *Richtlijnen voor het geven van injecties door verpleegkundigen in het kader van het Rijksinentingsprogramma*, Bunnik: NK, 1986.

Noordam, A.L.: Noodzakelijke aanpassing van de rubella-vaccinatieprogramma's, *Nederlands Tijdschrift voor Geneeskunde* 127 (1983) 4010.

OHE (Office of Health Economics): *Childhood Vaccination; current controversies*, London: OHE, 1984.

Oost, J. van: *Vaccinatietoestand van en inhaalvaccinaties bij een cohort lagereschoolverlaters te's-Gravenhage*, Leiden: NIPG/TNO, 1987 (scriptie opleiding Jeugdgezondheidszorg).

Poolman, J.T. & Rijkers, G.T.: Vaccin gebaseerd op het kapselpolysachcharide van Haemophilus influenzae type b, *Nederlands Tijdschrift voor Geneeskunde* 132 (1988) 1737–1740.

Quast, U.: *Hundert kniffliche Impffragen*, Stuttgart: Hippokrates Verlag, 1986.

Rey, M.: Le futur des vaccinations, *La Presse Médicale*, 19, 17 November (1990) 38.

RIV (Rijksinstituut voor de Volksgezondheid): *Vademecum 1981.*

Robertson, R.L., Foster, S.O., Hull, H.F., Williams, P.J.: Cost-effectiveness of immunization in The Gambia, *Journal of Tropical Medicine and Hygiene* 88 (1985) 343–351.

Rümke, H.C.: Evaluatie van het Rijksvaccinatieprogramma, *Nederlands Tijdschrift voor Geneeskunde* 133 (1989) 866–868.

Rümke, H.C. & Poolman, J.T.: Geconjugeerde vaccins tegen Haemophilus Influenzae type b, *Nederlands Tijdschrift voor Geneeskunde* 135 (1991) 4–6.

Schoenbaum, S.C.: Benefit-cost aspects of rubella immunization, *Reviews of Infectious Diseases* 7 Suppl 1 (1985) 210–211.

Schulpen, T.W.J. & Weerkamp-Wolfenbuttel, F.E.M.: De diagnose "kinkhoest"; een samenwerkingsexperiment in Overvecht, *Medisch Contact* (1984) 1615–1616.

Shephard, D.S., Sanoh, L., Coffi, E.: Cost-effectiveness of the expanded programme on immunization in the Ivory Cost, *Social Science and Medicine* 22 (1986) 369–379.

Spook, H.J.J.: Vaccinatie tegen rodehond, *Tijdschrift voor Jeugdgezondheidszorg* 14 (1982) 61–62.

Swaak, A.J.: Lokale klachten bij kinderen van de jaarklassen 1960 en 1961 na een herhalingsinjectie met DKTP-entstof, *Nederlands Tijdschrift voor Geneeskunde* 110 (1966) 332–334 (a).

Swaak, A.J.: Een onderzoek bij kinderen van de jaarklassen 1962 naar het verband tussen lokale klachten en de aard van de entstof bij immunisatie tegen kinkhoest, difterie, tetanus en poliomyelitis, *Nederlands Tijdschrift voor Geneeskunde* 110 (1966) 1696–1699 (b).

Swaak, A.J.: Enige gegevens over de immunisaties bij zuigelingen van de jaarklassen 1959 tot en met 1966 in de provincie Noord-Brabant, *Nederlands Tijdschrift voor Geneeskunde* 112 (1968) 889–891.

Veen, J. van der: Vaccinatie tegen bof en rubella; het advies van de Gezondheidsraad, *Nederlands Tijdschrift voor Geneeskunde* 128 (1984) 1150–1152.

Verbrugge, H.P.: The National Immunization Program of The Netherlands, *Pediatrics* 86 Suppl (1990) 1060–1063.

Verbrugge, H.P.: *National Immunization Programme in The Netherlands*, Paper presented at the 4th European meeting of National Programme Managers WHO-EPI (Expanded Programme on Immunization), St. Vincent, May 1991 (a).

Verbrugge, H.P.: *Persoonlijke mededelingen tijdens GHI/PAJ-overleg*, September to December 1991 (b).

Wagenvoort, J.H.T.: *Epidemiologie van bof in Nederland*, Utrecht 1979 (dissertation).

Weert-Waltman, M.L.: *Morbiditeit na mazelenvaccinatie; een onderzoek naar de ervaring van ouders*, Leiden: NIPG/TNO, 1987 (scriptie opleiding Jeugdgezondheidszorg).

Werkgroep Hepatitis-B-screening van Zwangeren: *Preventie van hepatitis B bij pasgeborenen d.m.v. screening van zwangeren op hepatits B antigenen en inenting van de pasgeborenen van positief bevonden moeders; Advies aan de staatssecretaris van WVC*, Leidschendam 1986.

WHO: *Expanded Programme on immunization; Immunization Policy*, Genève 1986.

WHO: *Expanded Programme on immunization; a report from the programme on communicable diseases; report on the second meeting of national programme managers on the EPI, Istanbul 1989*, Copenhagen 1989.

3 Screening for phenylketonuria and congenital hypothyroidism

Phenylketonuria (PKU) and congenital hypothyroidism (CHT) are congenital disorders which, if they are not treated promptly lead to, among other things, serious mental retardation. In the Netherlands, virtually all neonates are screened for PKU and CHT. PKU screening was introduced in 1974, CHT screening in 1981. The screening for PKU and CHT is a form of standardized programmed prevention. The aim of the screening is to detect the disorders at the earliest possible stage so that, through prompt treatment, the consequences of the diseases can be prevented. In this chapter, the disorders are described, then the organization of the screening is discussed. Subsequently, the effectiveness of the two screenings is looked at, and a cost-benefit analysis of each screening is made. Finally, a number of questions are raised in the conclusions, and the recommendations of the Project Group are given.

3.1 Phenylketonuria (PKU)

PKU is an autosomal recessive hereditary metabolic disorder that is caused by the virtual inactivity of the enzyme phenylalanine hydroxylase. This enzyme is the catalyst for the metabolism of the amino acid phenylalanine into tyrosine. The result is an excess of phenylalanine and its by-products in the body. This raised concentration causes irreversible damage to the central nervous system. Newborn children with PKU are clinically normal. The mental retardation and developmental retardation caused by untreated PKU may become visible after approximately 6 months, and will be obvious at the end of the first year. Therefore, PKU can only be diagnosed on the basis of symptoms or clinical findings when the irreversible neurological damage is already extensive (Avery & First 1989). A related (autosomal recessive hereditary) disease is hyperphenylalaninemia (HPA). 'In children with HPA there is still a slight to considerable residual activity of the enzyme phenylalanine. It is unknown whether HPA leads to clinical symptoms' (Verkerk et al. 1990). The number of children with HPA that has been treated is very small. Two other fairly rare variants (both called malignant HPA) are characterized by the lack of the co-factor tetrahydrobiopterin. This cofactor is essential for the action of the enzyme phenylalanine hydroxylase so that, also in these forms, the phenylalanine is not converted into tyrosine. 'The prevalence of PKU, treated HPA and malignant HPA among the neonates in the Netherlands was 1:18,000, 1:132,000 and 1:130,000, respectively; taken together this is 1:16,000' (Verkerk et al. 1990).

PKU patients and HPA patients, with a phenylalanine level of > 0.6 mmol/l, are treated with a special diet low in phenylalanine. It is a strict low-protein diet, supplemented by a mixture of amino acids (virtually without phenylalanine). Patients with malignant HPA are treated with tetrahydrobiopterin; a special low-phenylalanine diet is not necessary for this group (Verkerk et al. 1990). Although treatment with such a diet largely prevents mental retardation and/or developmental retardation, follow-up research of treated PKU patients has shown that their intellectual development is slightly below average in comparison with the general population. A working party has been formed to follow up the intellectual development of treated PKU patients (Verkerk et al. 1990).

3.2 Congenital hypothyroidism (CHT)

'CHT is a congenital deficient functioning of the thyroid gland that results in disorders of physical growth and development and serious permanent retardation of mental development... There are practically no symptoms of hypothyroidism in the neonate to begin with and what symptoms there are, are not characteristic of the disease. At birth these children are sometimes longer and heavier than average. After that the following symptoms appear: muscular weakness, striking facial features (broad, low base of the nose, oedema around the eyelids), large tongue, oedema, slow heartbeat, low temperature, prolonged jaundice, umbilical hernia and a swollen abdomen. Strikingly large fontanelles and late eruption of the teeth are signs of retarded skeletal development' (Schuil 1987).

'In principle there are three forms of CHT. In the most frequently seen form, primary CHT (approximately 93% of all CHT cases in the Netherlands), the cause lies in the thyroid gland. Primary CHT is characterized by the combination of low thyroxine and high thyrotropin values. In 1988, the prevalence of primary CHT was 1:3700 and in 1989, 1:2800. Both values show a great similarity to other Western countries (1:3000–1:4000)' (Verkerk & Vaandrager 1990b). In the other two forms of CHT, secondary and tertiary CHT, (together approximately 7% of all CHT cases in the Netherlands) the cause is not the thyroid gland itself, but the inadequate stimulation of the thyroid gland by the regulating centres (the hypophysis and hypothalamus). Here low thyroxin values are found while the thyrotropin values are not raised (Meijer 1984). In its annual report for 1989, the National Committee for CHT Monitoring (Landelijke Begeleidingscommissie CHT) (LBC-CHT) (Verkerk & Vaandrager 1990b) observes with respect to the prevalence of secondary/tertiary CHT that 'the number of patients with secondary/tertiary CHT is three, this is 1:63,000 live births. This prevalence is lower than that found in previous years. Vulsma (1991) and others report a prevalence of 1:26,000 for the period January 1981 up to and including September 1989. In addition to chance fluctuations, the fact that a significant proportion of these patients (26%) are not identified during screening plays a role.'

Treatment consists of oral administration of thyroid hormone (some-times lifelong), which causes all symptoms to disappear, except any brain damage that may have already occurred; this is largely irreversible (Schuil et al. 1987). Gons and others (1986), however, argue that recent data[1] indicate subtle abnormalities that are diagnosed later, also in patients who were promptly and adequately treated, particularly in the area of motor and perceptual skills, despite a normal IQ. These indications appear to be confirmed by a study of 28 CHT patients in northern and eastern parts of the Netherlands (Jansen et al. 1986) that showed that their mental and motor development was within the normal range, but that the average scores were below those of the standard group. It was also shown that half of these patients presented forms of neuro-developmental dysfunction.

3.3 Organization of the screening

The effectiveness and efficiency of a screening programme is partly determined by good organization, continuous monitoring and evaluation. Meijer (1984) gives a description of the organization on the basis of the following functions:

- The implementation of the screening is the responsibility of the Provincial Doctors Immunization Administration (Provinciaal Artsen Entadministratie) and, in Amsterdam and Rotterdam, of the Municipal Health Authority (GGGD) doctor concerned. The administration is carried out by the immunization administrations.

- There is a centralized system of quality control for the five PKU and CHT laboratories.

---

[1]Glorieux et al. (1983) and Jansen et al. (1986).

- The Netherlands Association for Paediatrics (Nederlandse Vereniging voor Kindergeneeskunde) has set up monitoring bodies for the two screening systems, the National Committee for PKU monitoring (LBC-PKU) and the National Committee for CHT monitoring (LBC-CHT), respectively.

  The LBC-CHT coordinates and evaluates the national screening for CHT. In addition to the LBC-CHT, there is a CHT Advisory Group (Adviesgroep CHT) (in which specialized paediatricians from the academic centres are the main participants) which advises the paediatricians who treat the patients about diagnosis and therapy; this group is also working on the medical aspects of the screening method.

- Continuing evaluation of the screening is carried out by the National Institute for Preventive Medicine (NIPG) together with the Dutch organization for Applied Scientific Research (TNO). These activities are financed under the provisions of the AWBZ (Exceptional Medical Expenses Act).

- Research on the occurrence of serious retardation in general mental, psychomotor and behavioural development, essential for the assessment of the effect of CHT screening, is made possible by a subsidy from the Prevention Fund (Praeventiefonds).

3.4 Implementation of the screening

The implementation of the screening is as follows: a blood sample is taken from the infant by means of a heel prick; this is done by the general practitioner, the obstetrician, district nurse, or by a staff member of the maternity hospital. The recommended age for carrying out this test is 6–8 days[2]. At this recommended age, 68% of children are screened: 4% are screened after the age of 14 days (Verkerk & Vaandrager 1990b). If the blood sample is taken earlier, there is a chance of a false-negative PKU result (insufficient protein intake), later sampling delays the start of any treatment that may be necessary. Immediately after the sample is taken, it is sent to one of the five PKU laboratories in the country. The phenylalanine levels of all the blood samples received are determined by means of the Guthrie test. The result of the test may be positive, dubious or negative. A positive result is an indication for immediate referral to one of the eight university clinics. In the case of a dubious result, a second blood sample is taken; if after the second sample the result is dubious again, or positive, this

---

[2] The date of birth is counted as day 0.

likewise is an indication for referral (Verkerk & Vaandrager 1990c). From the PKU laboratory, that part of the blood that is intended for the CHT test is sent to one of the five CHT laboratories. The thyroxine levels of all the blood samples received are determined. These are expressed in a standard deviation in relation to the daily average. For the lowest 20% of the thyroxine levels for a particular day, the thyrotropin values are also determined. When the thyroxin or thyrotropin values deviate sharply (positive values), this is an indication for immediate referral to the paediatrician. If the values deviate slightly (dubious) this is an indication for a second blood sample. If the result is dubious again, or positive, this likewise is an indication for referral[3] (Verkerk & Vaandrager 1990b). The number of second blood samples taken is determined not only by the number of dubious test results, but also by the number of inadequately filled strips of filter paper for the screening. This number seems to be increasing in recent years, particularly with respect to CHT. Verkerk & Vaandrager (1990c) conclude that this requires further attention.

3.5 Coverage of the PKU/CHT screening

The coverage of the screening is very wide: from 1986 to 1989 it was 99.73%, 99.76%, 99.76% and 99.74%, respectively[4] (Verkerk & Vaandrager 1990c). The reasons for not participating in the screening are (percentages for 1989): refusal/objection (0.12%), moved away (0.04%), and unknown (0.09%).

3.6 Effectiveness of PKU screening

Verkerk et al (1990), formulate the aim of PKU screening as the prevention of mental retardation. In assessing the effectiveness of PKU screening the following two outcome measures are the decisive factors:

- detecting and treating all children with PKU before the age of 3 weeks

- optimal validity of the screening method.

---

[3]In the case of premature children an alternative procedure is followed; this is described in section 3.7.

[4]Excluding children who died before the screening.

'The aim of screening, the prevention of mental retardation, is achieved to a large extent. Untreated, the majority of patients would end up in institutions for the mentally retarded and only 2.5% of them would have an IQ of more than 60. (...) None of the patients traced is living in an institution for the mentally retarded' (Verkerk et al. 1990). For the best results, the special phenylalanine-restricted diet should be started before the child is 3 weeks old (Avery & First 1989). All the PKU patients that were found in 1989 were treated with the phenylalanine-restricted diet before the age of 22 days, seven of the nine children were being treated even before the age of 15 days (Verkerk & Vaandrager 1990c).

The validity of the test is determined by the numbers of false-positive and false-negative results. On this basis, the sensitivity, specificity and prognostic value of the test can be expressed. For 1989, these measures are as follows: sensitivity 100%; specificity 99.99%; positive prognostic value 35%; negative prognostic value 100% (Verkerk & Vaandrager 1990c). The positive prognostic value of the test for the years 1974–1987 lies around 50%, in 1988 it was 68%, and in 1989 it was 35%. Despite the relatively low prevalence of the disease(s), the number of false-positive results is minimal.

From the start of the screening in 1974 up to 1989, three children with false-negative results were found. In one child, born in 1984, the disease was not detected until the age of 1.5 years, after her brother, born in 1986, had a positive screening result. The second child was a girl (born in 1988) with a negative test result, who was referred for further diagnostic tests because her twin brother had a positive test result (Verkerk & Vaandrager 1989c). The third child with an false-negative result was found in 1989. The disease was detected at the age of 18 months (Verkerk & Vaandrager 1990c). Verkerk et al. (1990) conclude that the screening test for PKU discriminates to a high degree. 'Assuming that the three children with an erroneous negative result were the only ones, one child is missed for every 53 patients found.'

3.7 Effectiveness of CHT screening

The aim of screening for CHT is formulated by Meijer (1984) as follows: 'to bring forward the start of therapy so that damage to the central nervous system is limited or prevented'. Since the process of damage to the central nervous system can start before birth and continues until substitution therapy (with thyroid hormone) is started, treatment should start before the age of 1 month, according to Meijer (1984). Gons et al. (1986) argue that treatment should be started before the age of 2 months. Finally, the report of the National Committee for CHT Monitoring (Verkerk & Vaandrager 1990b) states that when the screening was introduced the aim was for all patients to be treated before the 21st day of life.

In determining the effectiveness of the screening for CHT, the following outcome measures are decisive:

- bringing forward the moment that therapy is started
- validity of the screening method.

If we adhere to the desirable age for the start of treatment as stated by the National Committee for CHT Monitoring, the effectiveness of the screening is determined by, among other things, the number of children in whom the treatment is started before the 21st day of life (before 1981). For children born in 1989, that was achieved in 60% of cases (before the age of 28 days in 81% of cases) (Verkerk & Vaandrager 1990b)[5]. Before the screening, the treatment had started within the first 4 weeks in 20% of the patients (Meijer 1984). With respect to the effectiveness of the screening, Meijer (1984) also observes that 'on the basis of studies in other countries, it is highly probable that bringing forward the start of treatment as achieved in the Netherlands, will result in a considerable limitation of the damage to the central nervous system'. He goes on to say that, considering the age of the CHT patients found, both in the Netherlands and in other countries, a definitive judgement about the development of these children cannot yet be given[6].

The validity of the test is determined by the number of false-positive and false-negative test results. At the beginning of the nationwide introduction of the screening in 1981, the number of false-positive results was large; many false-positive results were found particularly among premature infants. 'This is because premature children tend to have low thyroxine values around the screening age (6–9 days[7]) without this being associated with a permanent form of CHT. Because the criteria for a "deviating" screening result of thyroxine were established for non-premature children, the screening values for thyroxine in a great many premature children were considered "deviating"... The thyrotropin values are usually not raised.

---

[5]In the report, the following (cumulative) percentages according to age are given (N = 69): 6% 0–13 days; 60% 14–20 days; 81% 21–27 days; 94% 28–41 days; 95% 42–55 days; 100% > 55 days. It was noted that, at the time of reporting, the starting dates of treatment were not known for seven of the children.

[6]See also section 3.2.

[7]The notation '6–9 days' could suggest that this means the sixth up to and including the ninth day; however, what is meant is the sixth up to and including the eighth day.

Opinions differ as to the meaning of these low thyroxine values and the desirability of hormone substitution' (Meijer 1984). For this reason, the criteria for a 'deviating' screening result for premature children (both those weighing $\leqslant 2500$ grams at birth, and cases in which the pregnancy was $\leqslant 36$ weeks) were adjusted. 'In these cases the thyroxine values are still determined and, for the lowest 20% of the thyroxine values, also the thyrotropin values; but in future only the thyrotropin value will determine whether or not further tests are to be carried out. Thus, as a result of this adjustment, those premature CHT patients who have a low thyroxine value and a normal thyrotropin value will be missed: i.e. the children with secondary/tertiary CHT, as well as some atypical cases of primary CHT (in which cases the thyrotropin value does not rise till later). Taking this deliberate risk of missing some premature children with CHT requires further scientific research' (Meijer 1984). The result of this adjustment in the screening method is that the discriminating power of the method is enhanced. Before the adjustment, 1% of all children screened were referred (Meijer 1984). In 1989, this was 0.49% (Verkerk & Vaandrager 1990b). In this group of referred children the chance of finding CHT (the positive prognostic value of the screening) increased from 3.6% (before the adjustment) (Meijer 1984) to 7.7% in 1989. This is still a low positive prognostic value: in order to trace one child with CHT, diagnostic tests had to be carried out on 13 children who turned out not to have CHT (Verkerk & Vaandrager 1990b). According to Meijer (1984), this number of false-positive results is considered justified because, as far as is known (practically) all children with CHT are detected by this method.

The validity data of the present screening method for tracing both primary and secondary/tertiary CHT for 1989 are: sensitivity 97%; specificity 99.58%; positive prognostic value 7.7%; and negative prognostic value 100% (Verkerk & Vaandrager 1990b). In addition to these figures, it should be noted that two premature children with primary CHT were missed (positive thyroxine values and negative thyrotropin values; according to the 'prematurity rule' they did not, strictly speaking, qualify for testing; however, the children were referred) (Verkerk & Vaandrager 1990b). The authors of the report comment that this number of false-negative results is probably an underestimate. 'Only after some years will a more reliable picture be obtained.' The report of the National Committee for CHT Monitoring for 1988 (Verkerk & Vaandrager 1989b) states that, in that year, three children with secondary/tertiary CHT were missed.

3.8 Cost-benefit analysis for PKU

Verbrugge (1983) concludes that, on financial grounds, PKU screening is definitely justified. The screening costs approximately NLG 2.5 million (based on 1981 price levels). This includes laboratory costs, the costs of vaccination administration, the costs of diagnosis and treatment, and the cost of evaluation. If the disease is not found at an early stage, most PKU patients will need prolonged nursing care in institutions for the mentally retarded. Verbrugge calculates these costs on an annual basis (including supplementary unemployment benefits) for 10 PKU patients, and comes to approximately NLG 20 million.

The Financial Review of Care 1992 (Financieel Overzicht Zorg 1992) (Ministry of Welfare, Public Health and Cultural Affairs) gives more recent data on the cost-benefit ratio of the PKU screening. 'The share of PKU tests in the cost of screening the neonates was NLG 820,000 in 1989. This includes laboratory costs, the costs of vaccination administration, and of the evaluation study by the NIPG/TNO. The salaries of the nurse, obstetrician and general practitioner, in connection with the taking of blood samples, are not included in this survey because these costs are included in the total care for mother and child in connection with confinement, and are not charged separately[8].' 'It is assumed that, if it is not detected, a child with PKU born in 1989 will become mentally retarded, on average in its tenth year of life (1999), will be admitted to an institution and will remain there for an average of 50 years (that is, until 2049). In 1989, the cost of one year of care in an institution for the mentally retarded amounted to approximately NLG 75,000. A period of care lasting 50 years would therefore mean a sum of NLG 3,750,000. By means of discounting, this sum has to be converted to a comparable amount for 1989. With a discount rate of 5%, the result is a value of NLG 840,000.'

'If a child with PKU is discovered by means of screening, then it is put on a diet for 20 years at a rough estimate, the cost of which amounts to approximately NLG 10,000. The total cost of NLG 20,000 is discounted for the period 1989–2009. Subsequently, a sum of NLG 125,000 is left. This sum has to be increased by NLG 82,000 being the cost of PKU screening in 1989, apportioned among the average annual number of 10 children with PKU that are detected. The result is NLG 207,000, a sum that can be compared with NLG 840,000, the amount required per child in the case of care in an institution. From this we see that the cost of a case of PKU that is detected early through screening amounts to 25% of the costs of hospitalization. To this we should add that this calculation does not take into account other relevant and often considerable costs such as benefits,

---

[8]In about 35% of the cases, the blood sample is taken by maternity nurses who did not have these families in their care, but were obliged to visit them. The district nurse cannot take the blood sample on her first visit, because that does not take place until the 10–14th day (C. van Riet 1991, personal communication).

loss of income, and such like. This weighing of costs and benefits has been limited strictly to those that come within the sphere of health care.'

3.9 Cost-benefit analysis for CHT

In 1984, Meijer made a rough cost-benefit analysis of CHT screening. He states that the annual costs of the programme for the health care system amounts to roughly NLG 2.7 million (including the cost of staff, materials, laboratory tests, diagnostic tests and central evaluation). As benefits, he formulates the costs that can be avoided with respect to the admission of CHT patients in institutions for the mentally retarded (at least four per year) (stay in a nursing home from the 5th to the 55th year; the cost of nursing care NLG 80,000 per year (1981 prices)). Depending on the interest rate chosen, this means a saving of NLG 550,000 to 1.2 million per unnecessary admission. Consequently, Meijer (1984) concludes 'that the savings effected by the programme are equal to, or even greater than, the costs of the programme. The programme pays for itself as it were...not to mention the other positive social effects of the screening (improvement of the quality of life, prevention of human suffering). Several cost-benefit analyses of screening for CHT made in other countries which, to a greater or lesser degree also try to take these effects into account, show an extremely favourable cost-benefit ratio of the screening programme.'

A cost-benefit analysis concerning the screening for CHT was also made in the Financial Review of Care 1992 (Financieel Overzicht Zorg 1992) (Ministry of Welfare, Public Health and Cultural Affairs 1992): 'The share of the costs of the CHT test in the screening of the neonates amounts to NLG 2.2 million. This includes the costs of the laboratory, of the immunization administration and of the evaluation study by the NIPG/ TNO.' 'It is assumed that a child with a form of CHT[9] that can result in mental retardation, born in 1989, will be admitted to an institution in its tenth year of life (1999), and will stay there on average for 50 years (that is, until 2049).' After discounting (see 3.8) this involves '...a sum of NLG 840,000 in today's costs per child. If a child is detected early by means of screening, the child develops normally as a result of the administering of hormone tablets. The cost of this amounts to NLG 100 per year, to which should be added NLG 250, the cost of annual blood tests. Taken together, a sum of NLG 350 per year, which at the end of an average lifespan of 75 years will amount to NLG 26,250. After discounting, this leaves a sum of

---

[9]In 10% of cases, permanent CHT results in mental retardation such that admission to an institution for the mentally retarded is indicated unless the disease is treated in time.

NLG 392,857, being the cost of CHT screening in 1989 apportioned among the average number of 5.6 children detected with a form of CHT that can result in mental retardation. Together this amounts to NLG 399,682, which can be compared with NLG 840,000, the amount needed per child in the event of admission to an institution. From this we see that the cost of a case of CHT that is detected early by means of screening amounts to 48% of the costs of hospitalization. It should be borne in mind that, in this calculation, the cost of the screening is only apportioned among the 5.6 "severe" cases of CHT, and not among the, on average 50, "lighter" cases, in which the prognosis can likewise be considerably improved by early detection and treatment.'

3.10 Conclusions

Screening procedures for PKU and CHT are good examples of carefully standardized preventive screening. The screening procedures are well organized, each year a careful evaluation is done, the screenings have a very wide range and, it would seem, a positive cost-benefit ratio. Nevertheless, there still appear to be some questions with respect to the treatment of PKU, the method of screening for CHT, and the false-positive results in screening for CHT.

3.10.1 The treatment of PKU

PKU is a treatable disease, but the treatment weighs heavily on both the child and the family. The National Committee for PKU Monitoring currently recommends that the treatment be continued for life (Verkerk et al. 1990). There are increasing indications that high phenylalanine levels are also dangerous at an advanced age. 'For girls there is yet another reason for not stopping the diet: children of mothers with high phenylalanine levels during pregnancy run a greater risk of intra-uterine impairment, the so-called maternal PKU syndrome. There are indications that such impairments can be prevented to a significant degree when strict dietary treatment is set up before conception and continued throughout the pregnancy' (Verkerk et al. 1990). In America it used to be recommended that the diet be stopped around the 5th or 6th year, but the result of declining IQs in children who had stopped their diets at around that age, has been that currently patients in America are also advised to continue the diet all their lives (Avery & First 1989).

However, there are indications that the PKU treatment may have serious psychological drawbacks. The diet is so strict that it could be questioned whether the negative effects of the diet are justified by the gain in health as a result of the diet. Research in this area is lacking (De Winter 1986).

3.10.2 The method of screening for CHT

There is as yet no consensus among experts as to the most effective method of screening for CHT. In addition to the method that is currently used in the Netherlands, there is a method in which only the thyrotropin value is determined. This method is used in most of the countries of Western Europe and in Japan, among others. In this method of screening, the number of false-positive results is far smaller, but the secondary/tertiary forms of CHT are not detected. In this connection, Gons and others (1986) observe that in view of the low incidence of these cases, it could be asked whether this is a significant disadvantage, the more because these patients will be detected on other medical grounds. Meijer (1984) observes that, in the countries where only the thyrotropin value is determined, the fact that children with secondary/tertiary CHT are missed is accepted. This acceptance is based on the belief that the mental development of these children will not be seriously affected. A further important disadvantage mentioned by Gons et al. (1986), is that those cases in which a delayed rise in thyroxin levels occurs will also be missed.

In the Netherlands too, a possible change of the screening method is currently under discussion. 'The present screening procedure can be regarded as an effective screening for primary CHT, provided action is undertaken in cases of deviating thyroxin values, and as a rather ineffective screening for secondary/tertiary CHT. If and, if so, how, the screening should be changed is currently a topic of discussion in an *ad hoc* committee of the National Committee for CHT Monitoring, which will report about a possible change in the screening procedure, and in the National Advisory Committee for CHT (Landelijke Adviescommissie-CHT). The most important question in this respect is whether secondary/tertiary CHT is a disorder that needs to be screened. In this respect, it is to be recommended that the criteria of Wilson & Jungner be used as a guideline' (Verkerk & Vaandrager 1990b). If this proposed alteration (present procedure, but only take action in cases of deviating thyroxin values) is applied to the data for 1989, the validity data of the test are as follows: sensitivity 95%; specificity 99.97%; positive prognostic value 54.8%; and negative prognostic value 100% (there would be one extra false-negative result) (Verkerk & Vaandrager 1990b). At the moment there is a proposal (trial project) to add a third test (thyroglobulin). The thyroxin/thyroglobulin quotient would supposedly have greater discriminating power for the interpretation of the result while a greater percentage of secondary/tertiary CHT cases would be detected early; at the same time, the number of false-positive results would drop sharply, so that fewer blood samples would need to be taken a second time (Verloove 1991, personal communication).

3.10.3 False-positive results in the screening for CHT

As mentioned above, one of the problems of the present screening for CHT is the large number of false-positive results. This is not only a technical problem in the screening procedure (validity of the screening), but also has emotional and psychological consequences for the families in which this occurred. In 1983, Tijmstra studied this and came to the conclusion that suspected CHT often caused tension and anxiety in the parents, partly as a result of shortcomings in the communication between parents and health care staff. Consequently, one of the recommendations of this study was that extra attention should be paid to informing both parents and health care staff. In the meantime, this has been improved. Leaflets about the screening are available for parents (in several languages). Whether or not these leaflets are adequate to remove their tension and anxiety is something that requires study.

However, a matter to which no, or practically no, attention has been paid, is the way in which general practitioners (in the event of a positive result), and district nurses (in the event of a second blood sample) convey the message to the parents. In the above-mentioned study by Tijmstra it appears that their communicative skills sometimes fell short on this point.

3.11 Recommendations

- It is recommended that the present situation with respect to the organization of both screenings be continued. The costs of implementing the screenings should be shown.

- With respect to the programme, it is recommended that the PKU screening be maintained in its present form.

- With respect to the screening for CHT a study is at present being done on a method that will result in fewer false-positive results. In this connection it is recommended that the present programme be continued in anticipation of the policy of the National Committee for CHT Monitoring (Landelijke Begeleidingscommissie CHT) (LBC-CHT).

- It is recommended that a study be done to find out whether the leaflets mentioned in section 3.10.3 are adequate to remove tension and anxiety in the parents.

- In addition, it is recommended that attention be paid to the communicative skills of those who are responsible for the screening in the event of dubious or positive results.

References

Avery, M.E. & First, L.R. (eds.): *Pediatric Medicine*, Baltimore 1989.

Glorieux, J. et al.: Preliminary results on the neonatal development of hypothyroid infants detected by the Quebec Screening Program, *Journal of Pediatrics* 102 (1983) 19–22.

Gons, M.H., Vulsma, T., Vijlder, J.J.M. de: Congenitale hypothyreoïdie; nieuwe inzichten en ontwikkelingen, *Tijdschrift Kindergeneeskunde* 54 (1986) 6, 164–169.

Jansen, B.J. et al.: *Klinische psychologische effectevaluatie van het landelijk CHT-screeningsprogramma in Noord- en Oost-Nederland*, deel 1 en 2, 1986.

Meijer, W.J.: Screening op congenitale hypothyreoïdie. Een wetenschappelijk onderzoek, *Medisch Contact* (1984) 15, 471–474.

Schuil, P.B. et al. (red.): *Nederlands Leerboek voor de jeugdgezondheidszorg*, Assen 1987.

Tijmstra, Tj.: Ervaringen van ouders na een vals-positieve uitslag bij de screening op CHT, *Tijdschrift voor Jeugdgezondheidszorg* 15 (1983) 6, 82–86.

Verbrugge, H.P.: Bevolkingsonderzoek. Fenylketonurie; screening van pasgeborenen een juist besluit?, *Medisch Contact* (1983) 31, 958–960.

Verkerk, P.H. & Vaandrager, G.J.: *Rapportage van de screening op congenitale hypothyreoïdie bij kinderen geboren in 1988. Verslag van de Landelijke Begeleidingscommissie CHT*, Leiden 1989.

Verkerk, P.H. & Vaandrager, G.J.: *Rapportage van de screening op fenylketonurie bij kinderen geboren in 1988. Verslag van de Landelijke Begeleidingscommissie PKU*, Leiden 1989.

Verkerk, P.H. & Vaandrager, G.J.: *Rapportage van de screening op congenitale hypothyreoïdie bij kinderen geboren in 1989. Verslag van de Landelijke Begeleidingscommissie CHT*, Leiden 1990.

Verkerk, P.H. & Vaandrager, G.J.: *Rapportage van de screening op fenylketonurie bij kinderen geboren in 1989. Verslag van de Landelijke Begeleidingscommissie PKU*, Leiden 1990.

Verkerk, P.H., Vaandrager, G.J., Sengers, R.C.A.: Vijftien jaar landelijke screening op fenylketonurie in Nederland; vierde verslag van de Landelijke Begeleidingscommissie Phenylketonurie, *Nederlands Tijdschrift voor Geneeskunde* 134 (1990) 52, 2533–2536.

Vulsma, Th.: *Etiology and pathogenesis of congenital hypothyroidism. Evaluation and examination of patients detected by neonatal screening in the Netherlands*, Amsterdam 1991 (dissertation).

Winter, M. de: *Het voorspelbare kind. Vroegtijdige onderkenning van ontwikke- lingsstoornissen (V.T.O.) in wetenschappelijk en sociaal-historisch perspectief*, Lisse 1986 (dissertation).

Further reading

Barnes, N.D.: Screening for congenital hypothyroidism: the first decade, *Archives of Disease in Childhood* 60 (1985) 587–592.

Brande, J.L. van den, Gelderen, H.H. van, Monnens, L.A.H. (red.): *Kindergeneeskunde*, Utrecht 1990.

Derksen-Lubsen, G.: *Screening for congenital hypothyroidism in the Netherlands*, Meppel 1981 (dissertation).

Hall, D.M.B. (ed.): *Health for all children. A programme for Child Health Surveillance*, New York 1989.

Huisman, J., Slijper, F.M.E., Hendrikx, M.M.Th., Kalverboer, A.F., Schot, L. van der: Intelligentie van vroeg behandelde patiënten met fenylketonurie; 10 jaar psychologische follow-up in Nederland, *Nederlands Tijdschrift voor Geneeskunde* 129 (1985) 44, 2120–2123.

Meijer, W.J.: *Evaluatie van de methode van de landelijke screening op congeni-tale hypothyreoïdie*, Leiden 1984 (scriptie vervolgopleiding Algemene Gezondheidszorg).

Meijer, W.J.: *Definitieve rapportage aan de Landelijke Begeleidingscommissie CHT over de screening op CHT bij kinderen geboren in 1985. Vierde verslag aan de Landelijke Begeleidingscommissie CHT*, Leiden 1987.

Ministerie van WVC: *Financieel Overzicht Zorg 1992*, Den Haag: Sdu Uitgeverij, 1991.

Vaandrager, G.J. & Meijer, W.J.: *Eerste resultaten van de screening op congenitale hypothyreoïdie bij kinderen geboren in 1986. Verslag aan de Landelijke Begeleidingscommissie CHT*, Leiden 1987.

Vaandrager, G.J.: *Eerste resultaten van de screening op congenitale hypothyreoïdie bij kinderen geboren in 1987. Verslag van de Landelijke Begeleidingscommissie CHT*, Leiden 1988.

Vaandrager, G.J.: Screening op congenitale hypothyreoïdie bij kinderen geboren in 1986, *Tijdschrift voor Jeugdgezondheidszorg* 20 (1988) 2, 19–23.

Vaandrager, G.J, & Verkerk, P.H.: *Rapportage van de screening op fenylketonurie bij kinderen geboren in 1987. Verslag van de Landelijke Begeleidingscommissie PKU*, Leiden 1988.

Vaandrager, G.J. & Verkerk, P.H.: Neonatale screening in Nederland, in: Es, J.C. van, Mandema, E., Olthuis, G., Verstraete, M.: *Het medisch jaar 1990*, Utrecht 1990, pp.310–322.

Verkerk, P.H. & Vaandrager, G.J.: *Rapportage van de screening op congenitale hypothyreoïdie bij kinderen geboren in 1983–derde meetpunt. Verslag van de Landelijke Begeleidingscommissie CHT*, Leiden 1989.

Verkerk, P.H. & Vaandrager, G.J.: *Rapportage van de screening op congenitale hypothyreoïdie bij kinderen geboren in 1984. Verslag van de Landelijke Begeleidingscommissie CHT*, Leiden 1990.

Winter, M. de: Screening en het 'wetenschappelijk ouderschap', *Kind en Adolescent* 9 (1988) 4, 266–276.

4 Screening for hearing impairment

Hearing is an important sensory function. The development of good hearing is of great significance for development as a whole and notably for speech development and language acquisition. Late discovery of hearing impairment may result in a disruption of development. At Child Health Clinics the hearing functions of young children have always been checked, but from the 1960s onward this has taken place systematically on all children by means of a standardized screening method: the Ewing test (Ewing & Ewing 1944). The aim of this method is to detect all hearing impairments at the age of about 9 months. In this chapter, normal hearing is briefly discussed, then the various types of impairment. Subsequently, attention is given to the problem of secretory otitis media (SOM) and its detection, the objective and function of screening and the methods of measuring whether or not the objective has been or is being attained. Then two other methods for the detection of hearing impairment used in the Netherlands are discussed and finally the recommendations by the project group are given.

4.1 Hearing

Sound is determined by pitch or frequency and intensity. Another distinction that can be made is that between tone and sound: a tone is a sound with one frequency; sound in general is made up of several frequencies. People with normal hearing can hear sounds with a frequency between 20 and 20,000 Hz and an intensity between 0 and 120 dB. Only a small part of the frequency range is needed to understand speech: between 500 and 4000 Hz at between 20 and 70 dB. At birth, hearing sensitivity is not at its peak, but it increases with time. This implies that a minor loss of hearing at the age of two may be far more serious from a development point of view than the same loss at school age (Bennet & Furukawa 1984).

4.2 Hearing impairments

Hearing impairments occur in various degrees and depending on their gravity may lead to deafness, or to serious or slight loss of hearing. It seems unclear exactly what is understood by deafness or hearing loss. Absolute deafness is rare; usually some remnants of hearing are left. The prevalence of serious loss of hearing is 1 in 1000 neonates. 'The hearing impairment may be confined to one frequency range (high, medium or low pitch) or may affect several frequencies. The extent of hearing loss may vary greatly, so for instance, soft sounds are not perceived or even loud sounds are not heard. Because there is such a wide variation in type, there is no proper classification of hearing loss in children. A classification into type (loss of frequency) or degree (sound level) is feasible, but has little meaning, because it would not do justice to the capricious patterns shown by many forms of hearing loss' (Schlesinger-Was 1986).

Hearing loss in children is of three types: sensorineural hearing loss (SNHL); conductive hearing loss; and a combination of the two. Sensorineural hearing loss is caused by a disorder of the inner ear or the auditory nerve, is usually congenital or acquired early and is permanent (in either stationary or progressive form). Conductive loss is caused by a disorder of the conductive apparatus. In the majority of cases secretory otitis media (SOM) causes the conductive loss. There seems to be consensus on the prevalence of sensorineural disorders: 1 in 1000 children. Little is known, however, on the prevalence of conductive disorders. The nature and gravity of a disorder are determined by the number of dB of hearing loss, the frequency at which this loss is manifested and whether it is unilateral or bilateral.

There is as yet little consensus on the measure (in dB) of hearing loss that is detrimental to young children. Bess (1985), *inter alia,* assumes a bilateral loss of 26 dB or over to be detrimental. Downs (1975) on the contrary, thinks that even a minimal loss of hearing is harmful to children. Little is known about the possible consequences for children of unilateral loss of hearing. According to Schlesinger-Was (1986) it is assumed by some, on insufficient grounds, that unilateral loss has little or no influence on language acquisition. Research by Bess (1985), Quigley and Thomure (1986), Boyd (1974) and Bess and Tharpe (1984) however seems to justify the conclusion that children can indeed be (temporarily) retarded as a result of unilateral loss.

To sum up, it may be said that there is no consensus on the degree of hearing loss that impedes children in the development of speech and language.

4.3 Secretory otitis media (SOM)

The big problem that confronts us in screening for hearing impairment is inflammation of the middle ear (secretory otitis media SOM). This disorder of the ear is one of the most common disorders in children and manifests itself as an accumulation of fluid in the middle ear, resulting in loss of conductivity. Paradise (1980) alleges that from the point of view of epidemiology little is known about SOM; aetiology and pathogenesis are only partially understood; the diagnosis, especially with young children, can be difficult, resulting in the disorder being under- and over-diagnosed in turn. Although SOM is common in young children, no reliable data for the Netherlands on prevalence and incidence were available until a short time ago. Results of research cannot be compared at an international level either, as criteria and measuring methods differ (Van den Broek & Zielhuis 1988). From the beginning of the 1980s Van den Broek and Zielhuis (1988) carried out a longitudinal epidemiological survey (the KNOOP[1] survey) among 1328 children between birth and the age of four. Before the age of four at least 80% of the children had one or more episodes of SOM; 50% had had bilateral SOM; SOM is most frequent around the ages of two and five years.

Little is known of what causes SOM. Many risk factors are mentioned, such as age, gender, race, genetic background, prematurity, congenital defects, socio-economic circumstances, season, infections of the upper respiratory tract and acute inflammation of the middle ear. Van den Broek and Zielhuis (1988) allege that out of all these risk factors the upper respiratory tract infection and recent acute inflammation of the middle ear are the major determinants for SOM. Analysis proves that the other factors jointly or severally make a minor contribution to the development of SOM. This means that there are no clear leads for primary prevention or for defining risk groups. There seems to be consensus on the natural course of SOM: in some 50% of cases spontaneous recovery occurs within 3 months, the chance of recurrence is also 50% (Van den Broek & Zielhuis 1988). Experts also seem to agree on the nature and gravity of SOM: it is a slight to moderate disorder which also concerns frequencies in the range of speech sounds and which although usually temporary may last a very long time. Usually the loss of hearing is between 20 and 30 dB but it may vary greatly in the course of the illness (Schlesinger-Was 1986).

A discussion about the consequences of SOM for linguistic development has been going on for years in national and international literature. The central questions are: is there a relationship between early otitis media and later impediments in language or cognitive development? If so, is this a causal connection and are these disorders irreversible (Paradise 1981)? Several surveys have considered these questions, with divergent results

---

[1]A research project carried out by the Catholic University of Nijmegen (Katholieke Universiteit Nijmegen Oor Onderzoek bij Peuters).

(Quigley & Thomure 1968, Hamilton & Owrid 1974, Keith et al. 1981, Sak & Ruben 1981). Most of these studies have the disadvantage of being retrospective and of involving only small groups of children, so that the value that can be ascribed to them is limited. Some prospective studies were indeed made (Kaplan et al. 1973, Silva et al. 1986, Van den Broek & Zielhuis 1988) which showed that SOM can have significant negative consequences for verbal skills (Kaplan et al. 1973) and command of the language (Silva et al. 1986, Van den Broek & Zielhuis 1988). According to Bess (1985) however, an unambiguous causal connection cannot be made on the basis of the present data. Paradise (1981) puts it as follows: there are countless proofs that impediments in speech, language and cognition of children are related to chronic and continuous disorder of the middle ear and loss of conductivity. It would seem reasonable to assume that the connection is, at least to a great extent, of a causal nature. The data at present available indicate that the lag in development is made up for when hearing recovers. There is no convincing evidence that a permanent lag in development may be the consequence of one or more SOM episodes during the first few years of life (or later), if at least no hearing loss has remained. But, conversely, there is no evidence either that such episodes are absolutely harmless to development. Practically all the authors mentioned consider further research in this field to be essential.

4.4 Aim and outcome measurement of screening for hearing impairment

There is some uncertainty about the aim of screening for hearing impairment. Everyone agrees that sensorineural hearing disorders must be detected, but there is less unanimity on the value of detecting conductive hearing loss (caused by SOM). Some authors think protracted (Schlesinger-Was 1986) and/or serious (Hall 1989) SOM should be treated and that consequently screening is worthwhile. Van den Broek & Zielhuis (1988), on the basis of the results of the KNOOP research project, arrive at a different conclusion: 'These results support current expert opinion that early detection of SOM by screening pre-school children will not have the effect intended (reduction of the occurrence of impediments in language development). Other data, notably those regarding the natural course of SOM, support the opinion that early detection of SOM in this age group is not effective and efficient... Due to the strong tendency towards spontaneous recovery and the limited influence ear tubes have on making up for an existing lag in language development, no clear net effect of SOM screening on language development may be expected.'

Even though the value of treating SOM is under discussion, detection of children with SOM (especially SOM episodes of 3 months and over) can serve a further purpose, such as informing parents about the temporary loss of hearing of their child and the possible consequences for speech development. There is consensus within the Project Group on the necessity of early detection of substantial sensorineural hearing losses in infants. The fact that this also allows a number of conductive hearing losses to be detected is considered a positive side effect. The Project Group is not unanimous, however, on whether the method should be suitable for the detection of all (protracted) conductive hearing losses.

In formulating outcome measures for hearing screening it was assumed that the screening should detect moderate to serious sensorineural losses as well as persistent conductive losses. To evaluate screening for hearing impairment the following outcome measures may also be considered (Van der Lem 1991):

- in regard to the screening method used (validity), for both sensorineural and conductive losses:
  — false positives: the greater part of this group will be found through diagnostic examination following the result of the screening
  — false negatives: it will be some years before missed children are detected. The type and degree of hearing loss has to be established by diagnostics. It will not be possible to find the group of children who had conductive loss of hearing at the time of the screening, except for children with a very protracted conductive loss

- regarding the consequences for the development of sensorineural losses:
  — the degree to which parents are informed with regard to deafness or (serious) hearing loss and the consequences
  — parents' competence in communicating with their deaf child
  — the deaf child's communicative ability
  — school results

- regarding the consequences for the development of conductive losses:
  — level of development of speech/language
  — the degree to which parents are informed with regard to speech and linguistic development and the consequences of conductive loss
  — school results
  — social skills

- as a final outcome measure for the two forms of hearing losses we might consider:
  — gains in health (sensorineural losses to be measured at the age of four; conductive losses to be measured at the age of eight or nine);
- as a final outcome measure for sensorineural losses we might consider:
  — wellbeing and career at the age of 20[2].

4.5 Screening for hearing impairment

The sounds (stimuli) used in screening tests, should meet certain requirements. During the Nova Scotia Conference on Early Identification of Hearing Loss (Mencher 1974) the 'National Joint Committee on Infant Hearing' recommended the prohibition of the use of sounds louder than 45 dB. Others, including McCormick (1988), state a maximum intensity of 25–35 dB. Further recommendations were that at least one high-frequency (2000–4000 Hz) and one low-frequency (500–2000 Hz) stimulus be used. Others are of the opinion that the stimuli should cover the range between 250 and 10,000 Hz. Finally the desirable frequency content of the stimuli is under discussion: natural, wide-range sounds or narrow-range sounds (pure tones). According to Sweitzer (1977) the natural sounds have the advantage of eliciting a more consistent reaction, especially from younger children. A drawback is, however, that they do not show up children with a specific loss of frequency. This condition is much better checked with pure tones. However, some scientists believe children react less well to these sounds (as being either not sufficiently familiar or not interesting).

4.6 Screening tests

Tests for hearing screening can be subdivided into subjective (behavioural) tests and objective tests. With behavioural tests the (anticipated) response is that the child displays some typical behaviour; with objective tests the response can be measured by apparatus. The advantage of objective tests is

---

[2]In 1976, a survey into this was made among young people who were deaf or hearing impaired. (Beroepen voor Slechthorenden en Doven: Occupations for the Deaf and the Hearing Impaired, Netherlands Ministry of Public Health 1977) (in Dutch). The results are comparable (Van der Lem 1991).

that the response interpretation is more reliable and the reproducibility is higher. The drawbacks are that these tests are many times more expensive (partly because of the necessary apparatus), that they may be more stressful for the child and that in most cases it is not feasible to carry them out in the clinic.

During the Nova Scotia Conference the Joint Committee mentioned above recommended that hearing tests be held at the age of approximately 7 months. All tests used in the Netherlands are behavioural tests focusing on the age between 8 and 10 months.

The test used most often in the Netherlands is the Ewing test (abroad too, it is the most frequently used screening test for this age group)[3]. Two other methods are used locally: the BOEL test (a test for the entire communicative capability developed by the Swedish Professor K. Stensland-Junker and named after the professor's daughter Boël) (Voorhoeve 1984) and the hearing behaviour questionnaire by Swaak (Swaak 1986); strictly speaking these are not screening tests. Schlesinger-Was (1986), after an extensive study of the literature, arrives at the conclusion that, when comparing the three tests, the Ewing test is the best as to quality, but that it requires a lot of manpower and organization. This problem is partly solved by the new version of the Ewing test (the Compact Amsterdam Pedo Audiometric Screener: CAPAS), which presents sounds digitally (making the test more reliable), is carried out by one person (a district nurse) instead of by two people (doctor and district nurse), and is recorded automatically. The new version of the Ewing test also meets the requirements of the Joint Committee with respect to the sounds presented: the stimuli cover four frequencies, namely 500, 1500–2000, 2000–3000 and 6000–8000 Hz.

---

[3]The latest data (Annual Report Early Detection Hearing Impairment; Jaarverslag VOG) put the range of the first Ewing screening at 86%. This percentage is influenced by the fact that in a number of places the BOEL-test or Swaak's hearing questionnaire are used. Institutes that use only the Ewing tests give a range of around 95% (National Cross Association (now National Association for Community Nursing and Home Help Care) 1989). If the child reacts inadequately to the first screening it is tested again after some 4 weeks (about 30% of the children originally called up); if this test is inadequate again, a referral examination follows (approximately 10% of the children originally called up). Should the referral examination be unsatisfactory, the child is referred to the general practitioner, who either treats the child or refers it to an ENT specialist. About 7.5% of the children examined (out of the total of children examined) is referred. Validity data on Ewing screening can be found in two surveys. One by Van der Lem & Baart de la Faille (1981) (with reference to both sensorineural and conductive losses): N = 34,252, sensitivity 79.4%, specificity 97.6%. The other by Baart de la Faille (1988) (with reference to sensorineural loss only): N = 54, sensitivity 95%.

4.7 Conclusions

The Ewing test is a relatively good screening method for the detection of hearing impairment in children about 9 months old. The test has good coverage, the validity data available present a positive picture of it. During the Project Group's discussions however the point was raised that the follow-up (after a negative result) often leaves a lot to be desired. Frequently, too much time elapses between a disorder being suspected and the diagnosis being made (and the start of treatment). In addition it has been mentioned that ENT specialists are not always adequately equipped for such problems. Van Plateringen (1987) draws the same conclusion. She recommends that better arrangements be made for registration, that specialists to whom children are referred be informed about the Ewing method and the action expected from them and that further research be undertaken on ways to improve the feedback of information on referrals. In reply, the Netherlands Foundation for the Deaf and Hearing Impaired Child (Nederlandse Stichting voor het Dove en Slechthorende Kind), which takes care of training for the Ewing test as well as its organization and administration, stated that they are drawing up a national referral protocol. Finally, a point that is stressed by many national and international authors: good, regularly repeated information for parents, in which the importance of screening is explained and which explains the significance of an insufficient reaction and of its repetition is of great importance. This will prevent much unnecessary worry by parents.

4.8 Recommendations

- At the Project Group's request, the new version of the Ewing hearing impairment test (CAPAS) will be examined for effectiveness and efficiency by means of the Erasmus University cost-effectiveness model. On the one hand this screening is a suitable test case for the model (because there are already many data available concerning the effectiveness of the Ewing test); on the other hand it will serve to determine the cost-effectiveness ratio of the new method of screening.

- It is recommended that screening for hearing impairment by the Ewing method be continued. On the basis of the cost-effectiveness analysis, the Follow-up Committee will have to consider, whether the programme needs adjusting, and if so, in what way.

References

Baart de la Faille, L.: Validity of large scale behavioural screening at 9 months. Paper presented at the EC Workshop on 'Early Detection of Hearing Impairment in Children', Montpellier, *Acta Otolaryngologica Suppl.* (1988).

Bennet, F.C. & Furukawa, C.T.: Effects of conductive hearing loss on speech, language and learning development, *Clin. Rev. Allergy* 2 (1984) 377–385.

Bess, F.H., Tharpe, A.M.: Unilateral hearing impairment in children, *Pediatrics* 74 (1984) 206–216.

Bess, F.H.: The minimally hearing-impaired child, *Ear & Hearing* 6 (1985) 43–47.

Boyd, S.F.: *Hearing loss; its educationally measurable effects on achievement*, Dept. Ed. Southern Illinois Univ. 1974.

Broek, P. van den & Zielhuis, G.A.: *Otitis Media met Effusie bij kinderen. Eindverslag van het KNOOP-onderzoek*, Nijmegen: Katholieke Universiteit Nijmegen, 1988.

Downs, M.P.: Hearing loss; definition, epidemiology and prevention, *Public Health Report* 4 (1975) 255–262.

Ewing, I.R. & Ewing, A.W.G: The ascertainment of deafness in infancy and early childhood, *Journal of Laryngology* 59 (1944) 309–338.

Hall, D.M.B.: *Health for all children. A programme for child health surveillance*, New York: Oxford University Press, 1989.

Hamilton, P. & Owrid, H.L.: Comparisons of hearing impairment and sociocultural disadvantage in relation to verbal retardation, *British Journal of Audiology* 8 (1974) 27.

Kaplan, G.J., Fleshman, J.K., Bender, T.R. et al.: Long-term effects of otitis media; a ten-year cohort study of Alaskan Eskimo children, *Pediatrics* 52 (1973) 577–585.

Keith, R.W., Cotton, R.T., Hoffman, K., Lawles, M.A.: Auditory processing in children with previous middle ear effusion, *Annals of Otology* 90 (1981) 543–545.

Lem, G.J. van der & Baart de la Faille, L.: Vroegtijdige opsporing van gehoorstoornissen, *Nederlands Tijdschrift voor Geneeskunde* 125 (1981) 2104–2109.

Lem, G.J. van der: Gehoor- en visusonderzoek (inleiding), in: *Effectmaten voor de preventieve jeugdgezondheidszorg*, interne publikatie Project Integrale Evaluatie Jeugdgezondheidszorg, Utrecht: Rijksuniversiteit Utrecht, 1991 (WP022).

McCormick, B.: *Screening for hearing impairment in young children*, London/ Sydney: Croom Helm, 1988.

Mencher, G.T. (ed.): *Early identification of hearing loss; proceedings of the Nova Scotia conference, Halifax, September 8–11, 1974*, Basel: S. Karger, 1976.

Nationale Kruisvereniging: *Jaarrapportage jeugdgezondheidszorg 0–schoolgaand, Kruiswerk 1987*, Bunnik 1989.

Paradise, J.L.: Otitis media in infants and children, *Pediatrics* 65 (1980) 917–943.

Paradise, J.L.: Otitis media during early life; how hazardous to development? A critical review of the evidence, *Pediatrics* 68 (1981) 869–873.

Plateringen, M.M. van: *Follow-up van Rotterdamse zuigelingen, die i.a.a. een gehoorscreening volgens de methode Ewing zijn verwezen*, Leiden: NIPG/ TNO, 1987 (scriptie geïntegreerde opleiding jeugdgezondheidszorg).

Quigley, S.P. & Thomure, F.E.: *Some effects of hearing impairment on school performance*, Springfield (Ill.), Ill. Office Educ. 1968.

Sak, R. & Ruben, R.J.: Recurrent middle ear effusion in childhood implications of temporary auditory deprivation for language and learning, *Annals of Otology* 90 (1981) 546–550.

Schlesinger-Was, E.A.: *Vroege opsporing van gehoorstoornissen in het kader van de jeugdgezondheidszorg voor zuigelingen en kleuters*, Leiden: NIPG/ TNO, 1986.

Silva, Ph., Chalmers, D., Stewart, I.: Some long-term psychological, educational and behavioral characteristics of children with bilateral otitis media with effusion, in: Sadé, J.: *Acute and secretory otitis media. Proc. of the intern. conf. on acute and secretory otitis media in Jerusalem, Israel, nov. 1985*, Amsterdam: Kugler Publications, 1986.

Swaak, A.J.: Opsporing gehoorstoornissen via gehoorgedragsvragenlijst voor ouders, *Maatschappelijke Gezondheidszorg* 14 (1986) 1, 26–29.

Sweitzer, R.S.: Audiologic evaluation of the infant and young child, in: Jaffe, B. (ed.): *Hearing loss in children*, Baltimore: Univ. Park Press, 1977, pp.101–131.

Voorhoeve, H.W.A.: Opsporing gehoorstoornissen, *Tijdschrift voor Jeugdgezondheidszorg* 16 (1984) 55–58.

Further reading

Baart de la Faille, L. & Kauffman-de Boer, M.A.: Ewing screening en de resultaten, *Logopedie en Foniatrie* 61 (1989) 85–89.

Barr, B., Stensland Junker, K., Svard, M.: Early discovery of hearing impairment; a critical evaluation of the BOEL-test, *Audiology* 17 (1978) 62–67.

Bellman, S.: Hearing screening in infancy, *Archives of Disease in Childhood* 61 (1986) 637–638.

Canadian Task Force on the Periodic Health Examination: The periodic health examination. Task Force Report, *Canadian Medical Association Journal* 121 (1977) 1193–1254.

Fiellau-Nikolajsen, M.: Epidemiology of secretory otitis media. A descriptive cohort study, *Annals of Otology, Rhinology, Laryngology* 92 (1983) 172–177.

Hall, D.M.B. & Hill, P.: When does secretory otitis media affect language development? *Archives of Disease in Childhood* 61 (1986) 42–47.

Hall, D.M.B. & Gardner, J.: Feasibility of screening all neonates for hearing loss, *Archives of Disease in Childhood* 63 (1988) 652–653.

Kaaijk, C.K.J.: Geleidingsstoornissen en leerstoornissen. Overzicht van de literatuur, *Tijdschrift voor Jeugdgezondheidszorg* 17 (1985) 42–45.

Lem, G.J. van der & Baart de la Faille, L.: Opsporing van gehoorstoornissen. Huidige stand van zaken en knelpunten, *Tijdschrift Kindergeneeskunde* 53 (1985) 113–117.

Melker, R.A. de & Burke, P.D.: Epidemiology of Otitis Media and the Role of the General Practitioner in Management, *Journal of Family Practice* 5 (1988) 4, 307–313.

Nederlandse Vereniging voor Jeugdgezondheidszorg: *Gehooronderzoek in de jeugdgezondheidszorg*, Utrecht 1991.

Northern, J.L. & Downs, M.P.: *Hearing in children*, Baltimore: Williams & Wilkins, 1978.

Rapin, I.: Conductive hearing loss: effects on children language and scholastic skills. A review of the literature, *Annals of Otology, Rhinology, Laryngology* 88 (1980) 3–11.

Stewart-Brown, S. & Haslum, M.N.: Screening for hearing loss in childhood: a study of national practice, *British Medical Journal* 294 (1987) 1386–1388.

Teele, D.W., Klein, J.O., Rosner, B.A., The Greater Boston Otitis Media Study Group: Middle ear disease and the practice of pediatrics; burden during the first five years of life, *Journal of the American Medical Association* 249 (1983) 1026–1029.

Ventry, I.M.: Effects of conductive hearing loss: fact or fiction, *Journal of Speech and Hearing Disorders* 45 (1980) 143–156.

5 Early detection and prevention of vision defects

The importance of normal visual development is generally recognized and therefore the significance of early detection of disorders in this development (such as squint and amblyopia, major refractive errors and serious structural disorders) is important. Vision defects that are unidentified or are identified too late may lead to (irreparable) impairment of vision, which can cause delayed and/or disturbed general development. Until a few years ago, there was no systematic method for the detection of visual defects that was workable in the clinic. Even though the Van Wiechen check-list[1] includes a number of items aimed at the assessment of the visual faculty, there was a clear need for standardization of research, evaluation of results, uniformity and promotion of quality and expertise in this field (Lantau 1989). To meet this need a standardized method was introduced aimed at the detection of visual defects at the clinic, Early Detection of Vision Defects (VOV: Vroegtijdige Opsporing van Visuele stoornissen).

In this chapter, the normal development of vision and the disorders that may appear are discussed. The significance of detection and the treatment of visual disorders is briefly touched on. The aim and function of the method of detection are then commented on, and some attention is paid to outcome measurement. Subsequently, the tests used in the Netherlands and some of those used abroad are described. Finally the recommendations of the Project Group are given.

5.1 The normal development of vision

Visual development is a fast and complicated process. At birth, the visual system operates at a low level; within a year vision has developed almost fully; the maturing of a number of visual functions takes another few years

---

[1]Partly based on the Denver Developmental Scale, the Van Wiechen check-list was developed in the early 1980s to promote the systematic examination of development (motor development, language and speech, personality and social behaviour) and to achieve uniform national registration. For details see Chapter 6, section 5.

(the plastic period). This period is generally taken to go on until the age of about 8 years and it is notably the first 4 months (the critical period) that are essential for further development (Loewer-Sieger et al. 1987, Campos 1986).

5.2 Visual disorders

Visual disorders can be divided into functional disorders and structural disorders.

5.2.1 Functional disorders

Squint and amblyopia are the most frequent disorders found when screening the vision of young children and may be the first sign of structural visual disorders (Boermans 1981, Gehrmann-Bax et al. 1981, Loewer-Sieger et al. 1987). Strabismus or squint describes a deviation of the position of the eyes, whereby the visual axes of the two eyes do not intersect at the focal point (Van der Hell-de Haas, undated). Squint can be manifest (a clearly visible and constant squint) or latent. A latent squint is not clearly visible but can be demonstrated when the cooperation of the two eyes is interrupted. Estimates for the prevalence of squint vary from 1.5 to 7% with an average of some 5%. Prevalence increases up to about the age of four (Bayley et al. 1974, Ingram 1980, Feldmann et al. 1988, Van der Hell-de Haas, undated). Because squint produces two different images the child will always use only one of the two eyes or one of the eyes will get preference (usually the one with the better acuity of vision). As a consequence the functioning of the other eye will decrease, possibly resulting in amblyopia. Amblyopia (the so-called lazy eye) is said to exist when the acuity of one eye has diminished without demonstrable structural causes, or if the decrease of the visual acuity is disproportionate to the structural deviation (Swaak 1978).

Depending on the age group, prevalence figures vary between 1.2% and 6.4% (Holt 1974, Bayley et al. 1974, Taylor 1987, National Counselling Committee for Early Detection of Vision Defects (LBC-VOV) 1988, Feldmann et al. 1988). In the majority of cases, amblyopia is found together with manifest squint (so that it is easy to recognize), but in some 30% the eyes are (apparently) straight (LBC-VOV 1988) Untreated amblyopia may lead to, *inter alia,* disturbance of central fixation on the retina, disruption of the capacity to see depth and severely decreased acuity in the suppressed eye. Refractive errors are disturbances of the optical system of the eye, such that a sharp image is not produced precisely on the retina. Little can be said about prevalence, because practically everybody has some refractive error; according to Hall (1989) the decision as to when a refractive error should be regarded as abnormal depends on clinical expertise and personal judgment.

5.2.2 Structural defects

Burgmeijer and others (1991) provide an overview of the defects that ought to be identified by clinical medical officers. Next to functional defects the following defects are listed[2]:

- congenital cataract; incidence 1:10,000 to 15,000; in half the cases the cause is unknown; known causes are hereditary defects or disorders during pregnancy (such as rubella)

- primary congenital glaucoma: high eye pressure; incidence 1:10,000

- retinoblastoma: (congenital) malignant tumour of the retina; incidence 1:10,000.

5.3 The importance of early detection (and treatment) of vision defects

The importance of early detection of visual defects is generally acknowledged. Most defects can be treated with reasonable success. In the case of defects which are not or are hardly treatable, detection is worthwhile because of the genetic implications and the guidance of parent and child. The most common arguments for the detection of amblyopia are firstly that persons with amblyopia run a greater risk of sustaining a disorder in the healthy eye[3] and secondly that in certain occupations ever higher demands are made on the acuity of vision of both eyes (Loewer-Sieger et al. 1987, National Counselling Committee for Early Detection of Vision Defects (LBC-VOV) 1988). In connection with the detection of amblyopia and squint, many authors not only stress early detection, but detection as early as possible. This is for two reasons: firstly a defect that has existed for a longer time is more difficult to treat; secondly central fixation is disturbed

---

[2]The defects mentioned have been selected on the grounds that a number of other authors (including LBC-VOV 1988) also mention them under detection of visual defects. A complete list of defects that can, in principle, be detected is not intended.

[3]This was found *inter alia* in research by Tommila and Tarkkanen (1981) in Finland.

more easily in young children. Therefore the results of treatment depend partly on the time of onset and the duration of the amblyopia. In the case of severe amblyopia, various ages are mentioned in the literature after which treatment is pointless, varying from three and a half (Ingram et al. 1986) to six or seven years (including Crone 1972). Obviously less severe forms of amblyopia have a better chance of a favourable result. The result, of course, not only depends on the duration of the disorder and the time of its development, but also on the treatment. There are different methods, of which occlusion (covering up the good eye) is best known and most often used. However, not everybody is convinced of the success of amblyopia treatment as far as amblyopia not attended by squint is concerned. Hall (1989) alleges that although worthwhile gains in visual acuity can be achieved, they are not always maintained, nor can the development of good binocular vision be guaranteed. Other writers, including Ingram (1980) and Stewart-Brown and others (1988) share this scepticism. All the same, many hold the opinion that the value of amblyopia treatment is beyond doubt.

A number of authors (including Ingram 1980, Atkinson et al. 1984, Neumann et al. 1987, Hall 1989), because of the scepticism about treatment mentioned before, take the view that attention should be focused more on amblyopia prevention. Notably refraction-amblyopia[4] can be prevented according to Hall (1989), Ingram et al. (1979, 1986) and Atkinson et al. (1984). Research (Ingram et al. 1979) has shown that specific refractive errors correlate with the development of amblyopia. By correcting the refractive errors these cases of amblyopia could be prevented (Atkinson & Braddick 1983). Ehrlich et al. (1983) however, are not really convinced of the correlation between refractive errors and amblyopia: 'Existing evidence suggests the correlation to be unacceptably low, leaving the door open for major under-referral rates'. They do, however, believe that the percentages of under-referrals in the surveys by Ingram and others (Ingram 1977, Ingram & Barr 1979, Ingram et al. 1979) ranging from 25% to 44%, are too high.

5.4 The aim and outcome measures of the detection of vision defects

At present, clinics in the Netherlands detect functional defects (amblyopia, squint and refraction defects), structural defects and visual acuity defects.

---

[4]In case of refraction-amblyopia one or both eyes have such a refraction deviation that no sharp image is produced on the retina (Wenniger-Prick & Loewer-Sieger 1988).

Everybody considers the detection of visual acuity defects to be worthwhile. The point of detection and prevention of structural defects is generally recognized as well. The first symptoms of these structural defects are often (in combination with other symptoms) amblyopia and/or squint. This being the case, it is logical and meaningful to detect these functional defects. However, considering the prevalence figures, the number of children detected on suspicion of a functional defect will be many times higher than the number of children that are found to actually have a structural defect. There is therefore a large group of children that have a functional defect only, with no question of a structural defect. Considering the lack of clarity with regard to the success of the treatment of amblyopia, it is questionable whether these children should be considered 'correctly detected children'. (This would also apply to squint and refraction defects, since these often lead to amblyopia.)

On the basis of the proposition that all defects should be detected, outcome measures may be formulated as follows:

minimum outcome measures:

- test properties:
  - false positives: these can be measured as far as functional, structural and visual acuity defects are concerned
  - false negatives: these are fairly hard to measure as far as functional, structural and visual acuity defects are concerned

- advancing the diagnosis: this is fairly hard to measure as far as functional, structural and visual acuity defects are concerned, but it can be done.

optimum outcome measures:

- health gains (result of treatment):
  - amblyopia and squint: outcome measure is the number of children having these defects at the age of 7 years
  - structural defects: determination of therapeutic effects at the age of 3 years
  - visual acuity defects: final acuity measurable from the moment of detection (3 years).

long-term outcome measurement for amblyopia:

- damage to the good eye in people with amblyopia (leading to blindness) at about 50 years of age (by means of retrospective research).

5.5 Tests for early detection of vision defects in the Netherlands

In the remainder of this chapter, structural vision defects are no longer treated separately, since the compilers of the method allege that the structural visual defects can be detected through the development of functional defects (National Counselling Committee for Early Detection of Vision Defects (LBC-VOV) 1988). Tests for the detection of functional defects will therefore also detect structural defects.

5.5.1 The Early Detection method

The Early Detection method is a systematized method of examination to detect defects of the eyes, their position and movement in babies and young children. Particular attention is paid to the position and the movement of the eyes. The method is not primarily aimed at the identification of acuity deviations or refraction errors (Lantau 1989).

In addition to taking down a short history[5] the method comprises:

- inspection of the eyes:
    - clarity and diameter of the cornea (*inter alia* in connection with high eye pressure with congenital glaucoma)
    - form and colour of the pupil; in connection with structural defects such as cataract and retinoblastoma
    - reaction of the pupil to light

- (ascertaining the position of) reflex images: in this way a straight eye position and manifest squint are differentiated

- cover test to confirm a straight eye position or a manifest squint and for the detection of a latent squint; the cover test acts as a check on the reflex images method

- following movements: these must be checked binocularly as well as monocularly. Notably the monocular following movements are important, as defects in central fixation, a feature of amblyopia at an early age, become evident in faltering following movements. These can best be established by comparing the left and right eyes;

---

[5]This history covers the following subjects: the mother's opinion on possible vision defects in the child, family history and the prenatal and perinatal histories.

the monocular following movements give an impression of visual acuity.

The examination is carried out by clinical medical officers (who are trained by orthoptists) with simple tools (a fixation light and perhaps a small toy animal) and, according to the compilers, does not take long. In a trial test in Amsterdam the time per child proved to be about 2 minutes (Lantau & Loewer-Sieger 1987).

Since the maturing of the visual system is a development process that for the greater part takes place in the first 3 years of life, the compilers maintain that the test should be carried out at diverse ages in the period between birth and four years. From the age of 4 weeks a first eye inspection should be carried out, viewing the red reflex, the fixation and the following movements, the clarity of the cornea, the form and colour of the pupil and the reaction of the pupil to light. From the age of 26 weeks the inspection can be done systematically (for organizational reasons this will often be between the ages of 7 and 10 months). In case of inadequate results, the child is referred to the family doctor and/or ophthalmologist. Systematic examination at an age under 26 weeks is not yet practicable with every child. The inspection is to be repeated at the age of 18 months. After that there is to be an inspection in the period between 2 and 3 years. Finally examinations from the age of 3 years are to be supplemented by vision testing (Lantau 1992, personal communication).

Two trial surveys were carried out with this method:

- 1975–1988 with 1200 children. The percentage of referrals was 4.5%; the percentages of false-positive and false-negative results were 45.2% and nil, respectively

- 1984–1986 with 5700 children. The percentage of defects found in infants was 1.6%. In this survey the test was also carried out at the age of 18 months when the percentage of defects found was 0.5%. The percentage of false-positive results was 55.2%.

The researchers conclude that in specific circumstances the method is quite practicable in the clinic and is excellently suited to be incorporated into the Periodic Health Examination (PHE) as a routine check. The clinical medical officers and nurses involved were positive in their judgment of the method, but made some critical remarks as well. Although the method does not take long, it is an extra burden within the time available for consultation. Some people also considered the organization and administration to be aggravating and/or unnecessary and finally, the dangers of over-medicalization were warned against (Lantau & Loewer-Sieger 1987). The Amsterdam Municipal Health Service has recently carried out research into the applicability of this method in its Pre-school Child Health Care. Results of this research were published in 1992.

Finally Early Detection has been the subject of a cost-effectiveness study (National Counselling Committee for Early Detection of Vision Defects (LBC-VOV) 1988). The cost of nationwide introduction and application of the method include the cost of implementation (notably the cost of training the clinical medical officers) and the permanent costs (including costs of training and guidance of clinical medical officers, working costs, costs of referral and treatment, and miscellaneous costs). In calculating two models[6], the cost per 'correctly detected and treated child'[7] is between NLG 200 and NLG 220.

The effects are considered to be:

- Promotion of the expertise of clinical medical officers in the field of early detection of visual defects. This constitutes an improvement in the quality of the Child Health Services.

- The Earlt Detection method can usually detect structural visual defects within the first year of life. This makes for a better prognosis for treatable defects; non-treatable defects can be referred early to Regional Centres[8] with their specific expertise.

- It will be possible to detect more children with amblyopia before the age of 3 years. Treatment before the third year will enhance the effectiveness of the treatment; this method will yield between 1700 and 2000 fewer people per year suffering from permanent amblyopia.

- Considerable costs, related to people suffering from amblyopia becoming blind as a consequence of trauma or other vision defects

---

[6]Based on incorporation of Early Detection in PHE with training as well as guidance by orthoptists (model A) or with training by orthoptists and guidance by district medical officers to be trained (model B).

[7]Considering the discussion around the success of amblyopia treatment, the question is, what a correctly detected child is: are the children with amblyopia, who do not have a structural defect, 'correctly detected and treated children'?

[8]The Regional Centres for the Blind and Partially Sighted are engaged in the assistance and rehabilitation of partially sighted and blind people of all age groups; they provide advice and counselling, education and information, help (information and advice), day rehabilitation and ambulatory guidance (guidance at home), intramural rehabilitation (day and night care) (Algemene Nederlandse Vereniging ter Voorkoming van Blindheid; General Netherlands Association for the Prevention of Blindness, 1990).

to the good eye, can be avoided. Costs avoided: NLG 88,830 on an annual basis[9].

- With increased life expectancy it is important to older persons that in case of one eye failing, the second eye still functions. This will allow the person to remain independent. The considerable costs connected with the care needed by people with amblyopia who become blind at an older age, can be avoided as well; Costs avoided: NLG 2,263,000[10].

- Other positive effects of amblyopia detection, which cannot be put in cash terms, are wider possibilities in education and choice of occupation.

A possible negative effect is also mentioned. This is the temporary anxiety caused to parents in case of referral (National Counselling Committee for Early Detection of Vision Defects (LBC-VOV) 1988, Lantau 1989).

5.5.2 Acuity assessment

At the age of about 3 years the acuity of vision is also checked. This is done by using an optotype card. On such a card there are symbols or pictures of either the same or different sizes. The method most often used in the Netherlands is the Amsterdam Picture Card (APC). On this card there are nine pictures of different sizes, which the child must be able to name. Not everyone is enthusiastic about this method. Feldmann et al. (1988) argue that the outcome is greatly influenced by factors unconnected with visual acuity, such as late speech and shyness of the child. In some places in the province of North Brabant the Hellbrügge picture card is used. There are 13 pictures on this card. Swaak (1978) has done a study on the effectiveness of this method, the parents themselves carrying out the acuity test. Of the children referred, 89.2% were found to have a visual defect; the number of false-negative results is unknown. The test had been unsuccessful with 5.2% of pre-school children. At present a new method, developed in Finland, is being tested for workability: the optotype card developed by the Finnish ophthalmologist Lea Hyvärinen (Hyvärinen et al. 1980). This method has some advantages. In the first place only four symbols are used, which even young children can easily recognize, and in the second place these symbols have been designed to meet the demand that in the case of an indistinct image they cannot be told apart (all four then seem to have the

---

[9]The text of the cost-effectiveness study mentioned does not make it clear whether this sum is 'per person per year'

[10]See remark note 9.

same shape). The reliability of this test (correlation of repeated measurements) is 0.94 (Hyvärinen et al. 1980). Loewer-Sieger and Lantau (personal communication) among others, are of the opinion that this could prove to be a workable and reliable method.

A comparative study was made into the use of three different optotype cards for pre-school children aged between 4 and 5 years (Ten Have-Fooy & Engel-Quaak 1986). Although the age group is just outside the scope of this project, the results may well provide an indication for the use of these optotype cards for those 3 years old and over. The three cards tested are the TNO Landolt card (to be used from the age of 4 years), the APC (to be used from the age of 3 years) and the card by Lea Hyvärinen (LH card) (to be used from the age of 3 years). The main conclusions are:

- The Landolt card is probably a good measuring tool, provided the investigator is well trained in carrying out the test and provided attendant circumstances are ideal[11]; in non-ideal circumstances the Landolt produces many false-positive results.

- On the basis of the above, the Landolt has been dropped, on closer consideration the investigators opt for the LH card, since the APC proves to be unreliable for acuity assessment for the second eye because of a learning effect[12]. The LH card does not have this drawback.

According to the investigators the LH card has the following advantages:

- The card is not or hardly susceptible to the learning effect.

- The investigator's objective interpretation is facilitated by the nature of the symbols: with the beginnings of reduced observation two derivative symbols (house and heart) fall away, with bad observation all symbols are seen as rounds.

- In naming the symbols the child can use both abstract and figurative concepts.

- If the child's vocabulary is not very wide it can still keep track of the four symbols.

---

[11]These ideal circumstances are: correct lighting of the card (500–2000 lux), correct lux on the child (⩽50 lux), quiet surroundings, good explanation beforehand, sufficient time available, motivated investigator, cooperative child.

[12]For a reliable assessment the child would have to come back a month later for the acuity assessment of the second eye.

- The time needed to carry out the test is a little less: 92 seconds for the LH card and 107.8 seconds for the APC. The explanation beforehand certainly does not take more time[13].

- The reading distance of the card is only 3 metres. This is practicable in connection with the ever smaller rooms that are available and it considerably reduces the chances of the child being distracted.

- The symbols are of equal value, in contrast to those used on the APC.

- There is also an adult version of the card. It has been calibrated, just like the Landolt, and has been found reliable. This provides a possibility for a better longitudinal acuity testing from pre-school age till adulthood.

- A smaller number of false-negative results compared with the APC.

Disadvantages of the LH card are:

- For the time being the price is high[14].

- Manufactured in matt, non-washable material. This reduces reflection to zero, but attracts dirt.

On the basis of these research data a similar comparative investigation into the use of these (or other) optotype cards for the age group from 3 years onwards is recommended.

5.6 Other detection methods

In this section some methods for the early detection of amblyopia, squint, structural defects and acuity defects are discussed.

---

[13]Here account must be taken of the fact that the children are totally unfamiliar with the LH card, in contrast to the APC card. This could be to the disadvantage of the LH card as far as time is concerned.

[14]It should be noted that this survey was done in 1986. More recent data are not available.

5.6.1 Amblyopia and squint

The methods used abroad for the early detection of amblyopia and squint are generally combinations of two or more of the four tests[15] that are used in the Netherlands as well (Bayley 1974, Committee on Practice and Ambulatory Medicine 1986, Canadian Task Force 1979).

Opinions differ on the reliability of these tests. The British Joint Working Party on Child Health Surveillance (Hall 1989) argues that the correct performance of these tests requires considerable skill. They therefore recommend, that, if physicians and/or nurses (working in Child Health Care) have to perform these tests, they should be trained by orthoptists. Ehrlich et al. (1983) also remark, partly on the basis of three studies[16], that the cover test is difficult to execute and that it is not a simple matter to detect small deviations using it. Stewart-Brown et al. (1988) argue that the programmes mentioned for the detection of squint (also in connection with the detection of amblyopia) can be criticized, on three grounds: the low effectiveness of the screening tests; the large number of false-positive results as a result of the cover test; and the slight effectiveness of treatment.

Next to the tests discussed above, Ehrlich et al. (1983) mention tests for stereoscopic vision (notably the Random Dot Stereogram (RDS)) as one of the best tests for the detection of amblyopia. When this test is used as an amblyopia screening test the basic assumption is that stereoscopic vision is one of the first visual functions lost through amblyopia. In the Netherlands too, research has been conducted into the use of such tests (for instance the TNO stereo test) for the early detection of amblyopia (Walraven & Janzen 1983, Tan-Tan 1988, Lie 1986); so far this has mainly been targeted at older pre-school children (from about 4 years). The study by Walraven and Janzen among 730 children aged 4–18 years (1983) showed the TNO test to have a sensitivity of 100% and specificity of 93% in regard to the detection of amblyopia. According to Ehrlich et al. (1983) such a test can also be used with younger children. They mention two surveys (Reinecke & Simons 1974, Simons & Reinecke 1978) in which the RDS was used with pre-school children. From these studies, it appears that the test is easy to carry out, is effective and that there is no problem in getting the children's cooperation. Considering the positive results with similar tests in other countries, it is

---

[15]Inspection of the eyes, (determination of the position of) reflex images, cover test and following movements.

[16]Köhler & Stigmar (1973), Romano and Von Noorden (1971) and Simons and Reinecke (1978).

recommended to investigate the applicability of this method within pre-school Child Health Surveillance.

5.6.2 Structural deviations

It is unclear whether the British Joint Working Party on Child Health Surveillance (Hall 1989) assumes that structural disorders can be detected on the basis of (detection of) functional defects (taken to be the case in the Netherlands with regard to early detection). Apart from this lack of clarity, the British Joint Working Party on Child Health Surveillance has recommended not to incorporate the available tests for the detection of functional defects into the core programme. This is because they assume that the skill needed for a reliable performance of these tests is not sufficiently available within the clinical staff (medical officers and nurses). The British Joint Working Party on Child Health Surveillance recommends that the detection of structural defects be restricted to inspection of the eyes, red reflex, and history (with reference to risk factors) during the neonatal examination; in case of doubt this examination should be repeated at 6 weeks. At subsequent visits, ocular appearance is looked at and the parents are asked whether they have any anxieties about the child's vision. The British Joint Working Party on Child Health Surveillance argues that many cases are detected by parents or other family members; besides, a significant number are found at the neonatal examination and finally some defects are found on the basis of risk factors. The effectiveness of the British procedure has not yet been investigated: it is not clear whether all children with structural defects are detected by this procedure[17].

5.6.3 Visual acuity defects

Optotype cards are used to detect visual acuity defects. Next to the cards used in the Netherlands (the APC and the Hellbrügge card), various other cards are used in other countries, for instance the Hyvärinen, the Sheridan-Gardiner cards, the Snellen E chart, the Ffooks blocks, the Stycar 5-and 7-letter test, the Sjögren hand and the Landolt rings. Within this group of tests a distinction can be made between tests for pre-verbal children and tests for verbal children. In tests for pre-verbal children the child is not expected to be able to name the letter, picture or symbol, but to point it out on a card in front of it; it has only to be able to match it. With some tests both options are possible; name or match. Another method a number of

---

[17]The effectiveness of the British procedure will be part of the comparative study into effectiveness, efficiency and quality of the Dutch and the British PHE programmes (see Chapter 8).

authors (including Hall 1989, Bagley 1986, Ingram 1986, Atkinson et al. 1981) regard as promising is photo-refraction (Atkinson et al. 1981). It does not require the child's cooperation, so that it can be used with very young children (from the age of 8 months). Not much time is needed and it can be performed by nurses, after training. However, this method too has a number of drawbacks. In the first place it requires fairly expensive apparatus; secondly eye drops have to be administered to eliminate the accommodation of the eyes (cycloplegia), according to Ehrlich et al. (1983) this may have unpleasant side effects.

Expert opinion is divided as to the reliability of the available tests for the detection of visual acuity defects. In a number of tests, a child may score fairly high by guesswork rather than seeing. In this context, Brant and Nowotny (1976) mention the Stycar 5- and 7-letter tests and the Ffooks blocks; Tan-Tan (1988) mentions the APC and also the Hellbrügge picture card has a similar problem. Research by Brant and Nowotny further proves that young children frequently mix up left and right, which has nothing to do with visual functions, but everything to do with the level of development of the child. With reference to the Stycar tests, Stewart-Brown (1988) remarks that they were developed as methods for use in clinics. Research (Hall et al. 1982) proves these tests to be unsuitable for screening purposes. In regard to the other tests that were examined in this study[18] scientists reach the conclusion that these tests produce a lot of false-positive and false-negative results. However, so they[19] allege, 'in well trained hands...it would appear that the tests can be used to achieve a reasonable level of efficiency' (Stewart-Brown et al. 1988). The British Joint Working Party on Child Health Surveillance (Hall 1989) draws the following conclusion with reference to visual acuity tests: '...there is no clear evidence that screening for defects at this age[20] results in a better outcome than diagnosis at school entry...Available tests are unsatisfactory – better tests are needed'.

5.7 Conclusions

At present, the Early Detection method developed in the Netherlands is being implemented nationally; about half (30–35) of the regional

---

[18]Sheridan Gardiner Letters, Stycar Graded Balls, Stycar Picture Matching, Hundreds and Thousands, Catford Drum, Matching 'E's, Kay Pictures, Beale Collins, Snellen, Ffooks, Leeds Picture Test and the Stycar Miniature Toy Test.

[19]Stewart-Brown et al. base their pronouncement on research by Köhler and Stigmar (1973).

[20]The words 'at this age' refer to the pre-school period; the British Joint Working Party on Child Health Surveillance recommend the testing of visual acuity in children at the age of about 5 years, which is the age children in the United Kingdom first go to school.

Community Nursing Service organizations use the test. Up to now the method seems to function well and to be cost effective. In view of the lack of clarity still existing regarding the desired ages for and the frequency of testing, the Project Group recommended that the method be again submitted to a cost-effectiveness analysis by means of the Erasmus University model. The follow-up of preventive screening should also be included in the test. After all, the final cost-effectiveness ratio is also determined by the result of diagnosis and treatment. This 'follow-up route' does not appear to have been very well streamlined in all places, anyway; often months pass by between a referral by the clinic and subsequent specialist assessment.

5.8 Recommendations

- In view of the positive results in other countries with tests for stereoscopic vision for the detection of amblyopia, it is recommended that the applicability of this method within the Child Health Services for pre-school children be further investigated in the short term.

- With regard to assessment of vision it is recommended that a comparative investigation be carried out. An investigation should also be carried out in the short term, into the workability of the various acuity testing cards for children of 3 years and upwards.

- It is recommended that the Early Detection programme be continued for the time being. The Follow-up Committee will have to consider, on the basis of further cost-effectiveness analysis, if and if so in what respect, the programme needs to be adjusted. In particular the health effects of the detection of functional defects should be given attention. Explicit attention is also required for more precise determination of the time and frequency at which Early Detection is to be carried out. It is also recommended that the effects at the level of health of the British Working Party on Child Health Surveillance procedure be taken into consideration.

- Finally, it is recommended that attention be paid to the follow-up procedure (diagnosis and treatment), with regard to both cost effectiveness and the course of the follow-up process.

References

Algemene Nederlandse Vereniging ter voorkoming van Blindheid: *Adressen en informatie ten behoeve van slechtzienden en blinden en hun helpers*, Den Haag 1990.

Atkinson, J., Braddick, O.J., Ayling, L., Pimm-Smith, E., Howland, H.C., Ingram, R.M.: Isotropic photorefraction: a new method for refractive testing of infants, *Documenta Ophthalmologica Proceedings Series* 30 (1981) 217–223.

Atkinson, J. & Braddick, O.: Vision screening and photorefraction – the relation of refractive errors to strabismus and amblyopia, *Behavioural Brain Research* 10 (1983) 71–80.

Atkinson, J., Braddick, O.J., Durden, K., Watson, P.G., Atkinson, S.: Screening for refractive errors in 6–9 months old infants by photorefraction, *British Journal of Ophthalmology* 68 (1984) 105–111.

Bagley, P.: Problems of screening and its implications to the orthoptic service in West Berkshire, in: Jay, B. (ed.): Detection and measurement of visual impairment in pre-verbal children, *Documenta Ophthalmologica Proceedings Series* 45 (1986) 351–356.

Bayley, E.N., Kiehl, P.S., Akram, D.S., Loughlin, H.H., Metcalf, T.J., Jain, R., Perrin, J.M.: Screening in Pediatric Practice, *Pediatric Clinics of Northern America* 21 (1974) 123–165.

Boermans, G.L.: Verwijzing op CB's. Deel 1, *Tijdschrift voor Jeugdgezondheidszorg* 13 (1981) 50–51.

Brant, J.C. & Nowotny, M.: Testing of visual acuity in young children: an evaluation of some commonly used methods, *Developmental Medicine and Child Neurology* 18 (1976) 568–576.

Burgmeijer, R.J.F., Boeken Kruger-Mangunkusumo, R.S., Fernandes, J. (red.): *Periodiek geneeskundig onderzoek. Een praktijkboek voor de jeugezondheidszorg*, Utrecht 1991.

Campos, E.C.: To what extent is it possible to quantify monocular or binocular visual impairment in pre-verbal children? Role of clinical signs and of electrophysiological and psychophysical testing techniques, in: Jay, B. (ed.): Detection and measurement of visual impairment in pre-verbal children, *Documenta Ophthalmologica Proceedings Series* 45 (1986) 372–374.

Canadian Task Force on the Periodic Health Examination: Task Force Report. The periodic health examination, *Canadian Medical Association Journal* 121 (1979) 1193–1254.

Committee on Practice and Ambulatory Medicine: Vision screening and eye examination in children, *Pediatrics* 77 (1986) 918–919.

Crone, R.A.: Amblyopie, *Nederlands Tijdschrift voor Geneeskunde* 116 (1972) 789–793.

Ehrlich, M.I., Reinecke, R.D., Simons, K.: Preschool vision screening for amblyopia and strabismus. Programs, methods, guidelines, 1983, *Survey of Ophthalmology* 28 (1983) 145–163.

Feldmann, C.T., Hogervorst, V.W.G., Smeenk, R.C.J.: Jeugdgezondheidszorg, *Huisarts en Wetenschap* 31 (1988) Suppl.12 54–58.

Gehrmann-Bax, J., Waele-Neefs, J.M.F.R.G. de, Vaandrager, G.J.: Verwijzing op CB's. Deel 2, *Tijdschrift voor Jeugdgezondheidszorg* 13 (1981) 51-53.

Hall, D.M.B. (ed.): *Health for all children. A programme for child health surveillance*, New York 1989.

Hall, S.M., Pugh, A.G., Hall, D.M.B.: Vision screening in the under-5s, *British Medical Journal* 285 (1982) 1096–1098.

Have-Fooy, E.S. ten & Engel-Quaak, S.: *Een vergelijkend onderzoek naar de bruikbaarheid van drie visuskaarten voor de gezichtsscherptebepaling van jongste kleuters*, Nijmegen: Katholieke Universiteit Nijmegen, 1986 (leeronderzoek in het kader van de opleiding tot jeugdarts).

Hell-de Haas, Th. H. van der: *Het oog- c.q. visusonderzoek op het consultatiebureau voor 0–4 jarigen* (PGO 37), Bunnik: Nationale Kruisvereniging, z.j. (Interne publikatie van de werkgroep PGO van de Nationale Kruisvereniging).

Holt, K.S.: Screening for disease. Infancy and childhood, *The Lancet* (1974) 1057–1060.

Hyvärinen, L., Näsänen, R., Laurinen, P.: New visual acuity test for pre-school children, *Acta Ophthalmologica* 58 (1980) 507–511.

Ingram, R.M.: Refraction as a basis for screening children for squint and amblyopia, *British Journal of Ophthalmology* 61 (1977) 8–15.

Ingram, R.M. & Barr, A.: Refraction of 1-year-old children after cycloplegia with 1% cyclopentolate: comparison with findings after atropinisation, *British Journal of Ophthalmology* 63 (1979) 348–352.

Ingram, R.M., Traynar, M., Walker, C., Wilson, J.: Screening for refractive errors at age 1 year: a pilot study, *British Journal of Ophthalmology* 63 (1979) 243–250.

Ingram, R.M.: The possibility of preventing amblyopia, *Lancet* March 15 (1980) 585–587.

Ingram, R.M., Walker, C., Wilson, J.M., Arnold, P.E., Dally, S.: Prediction of amblyopia and squint by means of refraction at age 1 year, *British Journal of Ophthalmology* 70 (1986) 12–15.

Köhler, L. & Stigmar, G.: Vision screening in four-year-old children, *Acta Paediatrica Scandinavica* 62 (1973) 17–27.

Lantau, V.K. & Loewer-Sieger, D.H.: *VOV: Vroegtijdige Onderkenning van Visuele Stoornissen bij zuigelingen en kleuters tijdens het Periodiek*

Geneeskundig Onderzoek. Verslag van een feasibility-study in "Apeldoorn" en "omgeving Tiel", Amsterdam: Interuniversitair Oogheelkundig Instituut, 1987.

Lantau, V.K.: Effecten van een gesystematiseerde onderzoekmethode voor het vroegtijdig onderkennen van visuele stoornissen (V.O.V.), in: Bos, M.W. & Winter, M. de (red.): *Jeugdgezondheidszorg in de toekomst*, Amsterdam/Lisse 1989, pp.59–65.

LBC-VOV (Landelijke Begeleidingscommissie VOV): *Vroegtijdige onderkenning van visuele stoornissen (VOV) d.m.v. deskundigheidsbevordering aan consul-tatiebureau-artsen. Kosten-effectiviteitsanalyse,*z.p. 1988.

Lie, S.L.: *Preventie van blijvende amblyopie in de kop van Noord-Holland*, Leiden: NIPG/TNO, 1986 (scriptie geïntegreerde opleiding jeugdgezondheidszorg).

Loewer-Sieger, D.H., Wenniger-Prick, L., Lantau, V.K.: Vroegtijdige onderkenning van visuele stoornissen, *Nederlands Tijdschrift voor Geneeskunde* 131 (1987) 2230–2233.

Neumann, E., Friedman, Z., Abel-Peleg, B.: Prevention of strabismic amblyopia of early onset with special reference to the optimal age for screening, *Journal of Pediatric Ophthalmology and Strabismus* 24 (1987) 106–110.

Reinecke, R. & Simons, K.: A new stereoscopic test for amblyopia screening, *American Journal of Ophthalmology* 78 (1974) 714–721.

Romano, P. & Noorden, G. von: Limitations of the cover-test in detecting strabismus, *American Journal of Ophthalmology* 72 (1971) 10–12.

Simons, K. & Reinecke, R.: Amblyopia screening and stereopsis, in: *Symposium on Strabismus: Transactions of the New Orleans Academy of Ophthalmology*, St. Louis 1978, pp.15–51.

Stewart-Brown, S.L., Haslum, M.N., Howlett, B.: Preschool vision screening: a service in need of rationalisation, *Archives of Disease in Childhood* 63 (1988) 356–359.

Swaak, A.J.: Vroegtijdige opsporing van amblyopie, *Nederlands Tijdschrift voor Geneeskunde* 122 (1978) 141–146.

Tan-Tan, K.L.: *Screening op amblyopie bij de jongste kleutergroep*, Leiden: NIPG/TNO, 1988 (scriptie geïntegreerde opleiding jeugdgezondheidszorg).

Taylor, D.: Screening for squint and poor vision (Annotations), *Archives of Disease in Childhood* 62 (1987) 982–983.

Tommila, V. & Tarkkanen, A.: Incidence of loss of vision in the healthy eye in amblyopia, *British Journal of Ophthalmology* 65 (1981) 575.

Walraven, J. & Janzen, P.: De TNO-dieptezientest als hulpmiddel bij de amblyopie-preventie, *Tijdschrift voor Sociale Gezondheidszorg* 61 (1983) 86–93.

Wenniger-Prick, L.M. de B. & Loewer-Sieger, D.H.: Scheelzien en amblyopie, *The Practitioner* oktober (1988) 917–921.

Further reading

Atkinson, J., Wattam-Bell, J., Pimm-Smith, E., Evans, C., Braddick, O.: Comparison of rapid procedures in forced choice preferential looking for estimating acuity in infants and young children, in: Jay, B. (ed.): Detection and measurement of visual impairment in pre-verbal children, *Documenta Ophthalmologica Proceedings Series* 45 (1986) 192–200.

Balledux, M., Mare, J. de, Winter, M. de: *Project Integrale Evaluatie Jeugdgezondheidszorg voor kinderen van 0–4 jaar. Literatuurstudies*, Utrecht: Rijksuniversiteit Utrecht, 1991.

6 Developmental surveillance

In the first years of life, psychomotor and neurological development take place rapidly. The development in these fields is characterized by its great complexity. Although insight into the causes and the course of developmental disorders is still limited, there is consensus that development and therefore developmental impairment can be multi-causally determined. Expressed in the terminology of the ecological health model described in Chapter 1, causes of developmental impairment can be found in physical factors or their interaction (endogenous causes), and in both behavioural factors (child's or parents' lifestyle) and socio-physical environment. The care system itself may also influence the disorder (exogenous causes). A gross motor impairment, for instance, can be due to a physical factor (e.g. a muscle disease), to a behavioural factor (e.g. too little stimulation from parents), or to a factor in the socio-physical environment (e.g. not enough play opportunities at home and/or in the neighbourhood). And finally, a factor such as long waiting times for referrals may aggravate the disorder or result in the therapy or treatment getting underway late (influence of the care system). From the establishment of the first child health clinics, major tasks of Child Health Care have been to give attention to children's development and to detect disorders in such development early on. In the past there were no simple Dutch tests[1] available for such purposes; children's development was followed and disorders were detected (as early as possible) by the 'clinical eye' of the experienced doctor. In the early 1980s, a tool was developed in the Netherlands for systematic and standardized developmental surveillance: the Van Wiechen check-list.

This chapter begins with a discussion on the theoretical background to the concept's development and developmental impairment. This is followed by consideration of possible outcome measures which will allow us to assess how far the aims of developmental surveillance are being achieved. Then methods of developmental surveillance are described, in particular the Van Wiechen check-list used in the Netherlands. Finally the conclusions and recommendations of the Project Group are given.

---

[1]Some clinical medical officers used Illingworth's 'screening booklet' (1973).

6.1 Development

Development is a very broad and complex concept. Its breadth is best illustrated by the great variety of operational applications found in the literature, such as behavioural development, personality development, motor development, neurological development and psycho-social development. The unruliness of the concept appears from the various theories that have been applied in the course of years to describe, interpret and forecast children's development. The main distinction between these approaches lies in the emphasis placed on the different conditions that determine such development. The following theories can be distinguished, in roughly chronological order: development models attributing prime importance to the constitution or to the environment (so-called main-effect models) and models attributing the development to an interaction of constitutional and environmental factors (interactive models). Nowadays preference is given to a transactional model in which development is seen as a discontinuous process, whereby constitutional and environmental characteristics affect and modify one another[2].

6.2 Developmental impairments

Clearly the great number of theoretical concepts lead to just as many descriptions or definitions of the concept developmental impairment. In the biological model, a developmental impairment is seen to be caused by constitutional abnormalities or disorders. In the environmental model, negative environmental influences are blamed; in the interactive model both factors may be considered to give rise to impairment. Finally, in the transactional view, developmental impairments are seen to be the result of unfavourably proceeding transactions (interactions) between child and environment, whereby the child gets insufficient or no chance to adapt to its world, and then to (re)organize and to (re)structure its world. It is assumed in this view that man possesses a 'self-regulating power' (Sameroff 1975). The breadth of the concept of development, as outlined above, constitutes an extra complication when describing the concept of developmental impairment, particularly in the framework of a transactional model.

Such a profusion of definitions and descriptions of this concept also

---

[2]See among others Knobloch & Pasamanick (1968), Sameroff & Chandler (1975), Sameroff (1975) and Rutter (1982).

make it hard or even impossible to pronounce on the prevalence of such impairments. Added to this, it is hard to establish the course of developmental disorders; some forms of retarded development disappear on their own, spontaneously, whereas other disorders only become apparent in the course of time. Thus the age at which the abnormality is established determines its prevalence in an age group. There is a rather broad range of prevalence figures in the literature: Campbell & Camp (1975) mention a percentage of 0.5, the National Committee on Early Detection speaks of 5–10% (in its first report of 1979), Rutter et al. (1970) estimate prevalence at 15% and Brandon (cited by Camp 1975) at 20%. Finally, in a study by Schlesinger-Was in 1981, which to some extent formed the basis of the Van Wiechen check-list, a prevalence figure of 3–5% was established.

6.3 Aim and outcome measures of developmental surveillance

The general objective of pre-school Child Health Care is to secure and advance health, growth and development. In the context of developmental surveillance this is achieved on the one hand by early detection of disorders (aimed at securing healthy development) and on the other hand by increasing the knowledge and competence of parents (aimed at promoting healthy development).

To evaluate developmental surveillance, the effectiveness of both the means mentioned above has to be examined separately. The following outcome measures can be used for this purpose:

- concerning detection of disorders:
  - number of correct referrals
  - number and type of referrals related to age
  - fewer behavioural disorders in the age of 1–4 years[3]
  - increased parental understanding of the individual development of the child

- concerning promotion of healthy development:
  - increased parental competence
  - increased parental knowledge about development in general
  - increased understanding of the individual development of the child.

---

[3]This outcome measure is probably hard to implement as 'behavioural disorders' is not an unequivocal concept.

However, since according to current thinking the development of a child is determined by the transactions between the child and its environment, the value of developmental surveillance is finally determined by combining the results of these two means.

6.4 Developmental surveillance methods

In principle there are several possible ways of examining development. The first method is surveillance, by which a simple test is used to divide the population into two groups, one with a high and one with a low chance of an abnormality or disorder. A second possibility is the regular examination of all individual children (generally called developmental surveillance), and finally the approach to groups of children at risk can be chosen. Up till now surveillance for developmental impairments has not been a successful undertaking. Although an untold number of attempts have been made to develop reliable, valid and efficient surveillance tests, the results have been inadequate on all counts. The most well-known, and most frequently reviewed, test is the Denver Developmental Screening Test (DDST) (Frankenburg 1967), adapted for use in the Netherlands by Cools and Hermanns (1977) as the Denver Ontwikkeling Screeningtest (DOS). Although the DDST is a reasonably reliable tool, its poor validity makes it unsuitable for surveillance. Particularly for this reason, its use in such tests has been advised against. For instance the report by the British Joint Working Party on Child Health Surveillance (Hall 1989). Dworkin (1989) also stated that there were neither theoretical nor practical arguments that would justify routine use of a surveillance test for all children. One of the main reasons for the failure of surveillance tests for development probably lies in the complexity of the problem being investigated. Surveillance can only be successful when it concerns simple, stable forms of retardation or pathology. In the detection of developmental impairments, the problems concerned are dynamic, are not stable in time and moreover are extremely diverse in nature.

Although there is consensus in national and international scientific literature on the necessity of individual developmental surveillance – with eminent authors such as Frankenburg (e.g. 1975), Illingworth (e.g. 1971), Drillien & Drummond (e.g. 1983), Hall (1989) and Dworkin (1989) defending its importance in the context of Early Detection – there is less agreement on the way in which such surveillance should be carried out, and how often. For instance, the British Joint Working Party on Child Health Surveillance (Hall 1989) recommends a schedule of appointments of eight medical encounters in the age group from birth to 5 years of age, while advising against both routine use of surveillance tests and routine carrying out of developmental examinations. It lays emphasis on anamnesis, observation and the importance of information (on cares and worries) from parents. In contrast, the American Association of Pediatrics (AAP 1988) recommends a schedule of appointments of 12 times in the period from birth to 5 years of age, focused on history and appropriate physical examination. Although these programmes differ in method and frequency, the term developmental surveillance is used in both cases[4].

In the 1970s, experiments were carried out, particularly in England, with the risk group approach (among others Greenhalgh 1981). This should have produced financial advantages; after all, the entire population of children no longer had to be screened, but only those children who belonged to a group previously defined as being at risk. However, it was precisely the definition of groups at risk in advance (for instance in the form of at-risk registers) that resulted in the failure of the approach. Studies by, among others, Knox & Mahon (1970) and Greenhalgh (1981) proved the effectiveness to be very low.

6.5 Developmental surveillance in the Netherlands

In the Netherlands, developmental surveillance in the pre-school age group is carried out with the aid of the Van Wiechen check-list developed in the early 1980s (Schlesinger-Was 1981, Van Wiechen working party 1983). The aim of the check-list is:

- promoting systematic examination of development
  — for the guidance of normal development
  — for early detection of deviations in development and of pathological development
- achieving uniform national registration, enabling transfer of the data, which is a condition for longitudinal counselling in pre-school Child Health Care.

The developmental characteristics applied in the check-list were chosen

---

[4]Butler (1989) gives extensive consideration to the lack of standardization in the use of this term: in fact, 'developmental surveillance', 'child health surveillance' and 'surveillance' are used alongside one another. In one publication 'developmental surveillance' indicates the totality of all activities in child health surveillance, whereas in another the term is reserved for what in the Netherlands is called developmental surveillance.

from publications by, among others, Gesell[5], who has divided the developmental process of young children into five development fields:

- gross motor competence

- fine motor competence (eye–hand coordination)

- adaptation (use of the motor function in daily life)

- speech and language (all the ways in which a child communicates with its surroundings)

- personality and social behaviour.

The Van Wiechen check-list consists of two parts:

- the baby check-list (birth to 15 months) comprises 37 items divided over seven surveillance sessions (1, 2, 3, 6, 9, 12 and 15 months)

- the pre-school check-list (18–54 months) comprises 39 items divided over six surveillance sessions (1.5 years, 2 years, 2.5 years, 3 years, 3 years and 9 months, and 4.5 years).

The choice of age for the surveillance sessions was determined by what (in the opinion of the designers of the check-list) appeared to be feasible in pre-school Child Health Care practice, and was adapted to the most common frequency of and intervals between attendances. In practice, development surveillance is a part of the periodic health examination (PHE). Classification in surveillance sessions of the current check-list can be a problem when the frequency and/or age at which surveillance takes place is changed. In principle it is possible to adjust the check-list to any ages on the basis of the study by Schlesinger-Was (1981). In the check-list the aim has been to cover all five development fields in each session. The basic assumptions here were that abnormalities may occur simultaneously in several fields, and that an abnormality which is originally restricted to one field may eventually have an effect in the others. The baby check-list differs slightly in structure from the pre-school check-list in that other aspects of development come to the fore in the 1–4 year age group. In the baby list emphasis is on the gross motor system and in the pre-school list it is on fine motor activity, adaptation, speech/language development and social skills.

The Van Wiechen check-list also includes a parent registration card, kept in the 'Growth Book'[6]. The idea behind this is that parents are the most

---

[5]See among others Gesell and Amatruda (1974), Illingworth (1972).

[6]The 'Growth Book' has been issued to all parents of new-born babies in the Netherlands since 1978. It aims to give parents the information to help them care for and raise their children. For further details see section 10.1.2.

obvious people to provide information about the development of their children. Moreover, in this way, parents are involved in following this development.

The Van Wiechen check-list is not specifically based on a theoretical model about development and developmental impairments. In the check-list manual (Van Wiechen Working Party 1983) a developmental impairment (for want of an unequivocal definition) is described as follows: 'Development is a ripening process of the central nervous system and the senses. A developmental impairment is the result of a disturbance of this process, manifested by a different progress in functioning to that expected. What must be understood by "normal" or "expected" depends on culture, socio-economic circumstances, the child's sex, the constellation of the family or home environment, the physical environment (town or country) and on many other factors. Thus the child's situation at the time that its development is screened must not differ too much from the situation in which what is considered "normal" was determined. This is resolved in the new check-list by making as much use as possible of the reference values established at child health clinics for healthy children' (Schlesinger-Was 1981) (Van Wiechen Working Party 1983). A later addition stated that assessment of development may never take place solely on the basis of the Van Wiechen check-list but must also take account of the following:

- rate and stability of development
- presence of neuro-pathological symptoms
- the current condition of the child, as apparent from the general impression, the general physical examination and the biometric data
- the impressions of the parents
- family and interval histories
- occurrence of risk factors in the prenatal, perinatal and postnatal periods and in family history
- the impressions obtained by the clinical medical officer and nurse.

Such an integration of developmental surveillance in a total assessment of a child does justice to the transactional view on development.

The reference values used in the check-list were drawn up on the basis of observations of children at child health clinics. Items were chosen in such a way that 90% of the normal healthy children that visit the clinic demonstrate the characteristic at the reference value age. Thus the Van Wiechen check-list does not indicate a clear aetiological, pathogenetically described developmental impairment, but a deviation from average values. This deviation may be a reason for referral, but must always be seen in relation to the quality of the execution of the item and the integral assessment of the child.

Up till now there has been no explicit study into the effectiveness and efficiency of the Van Wiechen check-list. The use of the check-list in practice has been investigated (among others by Wilbrink-Griffioen & Van Eyck 1989)[7]. The major conclusions of Wilbrink-Griffioen & Van Eyck's study are that the check-list (and particularly the baby check-list) is appreciated by a great majority of doctors as being an aid in following development, but that a number of hindrances to its use have been noted:

- A great number of doctors had difficulty in eliciting and interpreting a number of items, so that development surveillance took a lot of time.

- Because the restricted registration possibilities of the check-list were found unsatisfactory, many doctors used their own registration methods; this hindered the transfer and interpretation of data.

- Use of the check-list proved difficult with children from ethnic groups, owing to a language and communication problem and because the list is standardized for Dutch children.

- Finally there proved to be doubts about the value of the check-list for the detection of disorders; many clinical medical officers had the impression that the disorders that they found using the check-list would also have come to light without it.

6.6 Conclusions

The objective of the study of development cannot be unequivocally described, partly because of the lack of generally accepted definitions of development and developmental impairment. Therefore it is not clear in advance what research on outcome must be aimed at. A number of developmental characteristics are employed in the Van Wiechen check-list;

---

[7]Chatab (1989) studied the application of the Van Wiechen check-list. It appeared from the study that the check-list was not suitable for standardized application. However, it is questionable whether such a conclusion may be drawn on the basis of this study. It was a cross-sectional investigation (one point of time at which measurements are taken) which may have given some distortion, particularly in regard to age-linked care.

this standardization is profitable and makes evaluation and quality control possible. However, its value in regard to health has not been established; to do this a cost-effectiveness analysis must be carried out. In preparation for the execution of such an analysis the Netherlands Institute for Preventive Medicine/Organization for Applied Scientific Research (NIPG/TNO), at the instigation of the Working Party, carried out a study on the identifying function of the check-list and on the application of the check-list in practice. The study is based on the data collected in the Social Medical Survey of Children attending Child Health Clinics (Sociaal Medisch Onderzoek Consultatiebureaukinderen SMOCK) by NIPG/TNO (Herngreen et al. 1986, Reerink 1989).

The key questions are:

- Are the item reference values established in the Schlesinger-Was study (1981) in conformity with what is found in child health clinic practice?

- Are there items which are frequently omitted?

- Are there, in regard to the score of certain items, considerable differences between the participating child health clinics, which cannot be explained by possible differences in the composition of the group investigated?

- What proportion of the children attending the clinic are referred before the age of two in connection with a possible developmental impairment, and how does this compare with the number of children known from the literature to have such an impairment?

It should be noted here that the extent to which the Van Wiechen check-list has contributed to referral decisions could not be verified. The check-list is not intended to be a screening instrument and thus no criteria were drawn up as to when a child should be referred. What could be investigated was which items pertaining to those referred were (repeatedly) abnormal in relation to the original reference values. The proposal for the study also formulates the anticipated results and applications, as well as the policy relevance as outlined below.

- A comparison of the frequency distribution of the items of the Van Wiechen check-list up to the age of two that were collected in the SMOCK study with those of the Schlesinger-Was study. Should there be clinically relevant discrepancies between the original reference values and the references found in this study, adjustment would have to be considered. After all, when establishing the references it is essential that the measuring tool be used in the way in which it will later be applied in practice (Bezemer 1981). The SMOCK study approaches practice more nearly than the earlier Schlesinger-Was study.

- The frequency of non-coding (registration) of an item. Items which are frequently not coded are apparently difficult to fit into the regular PHE. Their omission should be considered.

- A comparison of the percentage of referrals on the basis of abnormal psychomotor development with the percentage that might be expected on the basis of the literature. This will give an indication whether there is possibly an excessively high number of referrals in relation to the expected prevalence (over-referral). An attempt will be made to obtain a more accurate impression of the value for prognosis by checking the diagnoses of the referred children. Although the final diagnosis is not included as a separate question in the check-list, the preliminary impression from the material now available is that it is known for a great proportion of the children.

The real effectiveness, or cost effectiveness, of standardized developmental surveillance at the child health clinics can only be reliably measured by a longitudinal study. But such an investigation is a lengthy one and therefore a costly matter. The retrospective study at present being carried out by the NIPG/TNO on the basis of the SMOCK data will however provide further insight into the method of application and the prediction value of the Van Wiechen check-list.

6.7 Recommendations

- The Follow-Up Committee should establish, in consultation with potential financiers, whether longitudinal outcome research is required in order to draw policy conclusions regarding maintaining the Van Wiechen check-list. This should be done on the basis of the NIPG/TNO study and of the Erasmus University study into the possibilities for cost-effectiveness research in pre-school Child Health Care.

- Since both the NIPG/TNO study and the Erasmus University study provide an insight only into the identifying function of the check-list and into the method of its application, the health promotion function should also be taken into consideration in the final decision-making on the Van Wiechen check-list.

References

AAP (American Academy of Pediatrics, Committee on Practice and Ambulatory Medicine): Recommendations for preventive pediatric care, *Pediatrics* 81 (1988) 466.

Bezemer, P.D.: *Referentiewaarden; een verkenning van methoden voor het bepalen van 'normale waarden'*, Bleiswijk 1981 (dissertation).

Butler, J.R.: *Child Health Surveillance in Primary Care. A critical review*, London 1989.

Camp, B.W.: Introduction, in: Frankenburg, W.K., Camp, B.W. (eds.): *Pediatric screening tests*, Springfield, Ill: C.C. Thomas, 1975.

Campbell, W.D. & Camp, B.W.: Developmental screening, in: Frankenburg, W.K., Camp, B.W. (eds.): *Pediatric screening tests*, Springfield, Ill: C.C. Thomas, 1975.

Chatab, J.: *Consultatiebureau-teams in beeld: een onderzoek naar de zorg voor zuigelingen en kleuters*, Utrecht 1989.

Cools, A.T.M. & Hermanns, J.M.A.: Vroegtijdige onderkenning van problemen in de ontwikkeling van kinderen. Lisse: Swets & Zeitlinger, 1977 (dissertation).

Drillien, C.M. & Drummond, M.B.: *Developmental Screening and the Child with Special Needs; A Population Study of 5000 Children (= Clinics in Developmental Medicine No.86)*, London/Philadelphia 1983.

Dworkin, P.H.: Developmental Screening – Expecting the Impossible?, *Pediatrics* 83 (1989) 4, 619–622.

Frankenburg, W.K. & Dodds, J.B.: The Denver Developmental Screening Test, *Journal of Pediatrics* 71 (1967) 181–191.

Greenhalgh, P.M.: *Why developmental screening*, Oxford 1981.

Hall, D.M.B. (ed.): *Health for All Children. A Programme for Child Health Surveillance*, New York 1989.

Herngreen, W.P., Noord-Zaadstra, B.M. van, Schlesinger-Was, E.A.: Longitudinale referentiegegevens met betrekking tot groei, ontwikkeling en morbiditeit gedurende de eerste twee levensjaren, *Tijdschrift Sociale Gezondheidszorg* 64 (1986) 544–546.

Horowitz, F.D. (ed.): *Review of child development. Vol. 4*, Chicago 1975.

Illingworth, R.S.: The predictive value of developmental assessment in infancy, *Developmental Medicine and Child Neurology* 13 (1971) 721–725.

Illingworth, R.S.: *The development of the infant and young child, normal and abnormal*, Edinburgh 1972.

Illingworth, R.S.: *Basic developmental screening 0–2 years*, London: Blackwell, 1973.

Knobloch, H. & Pasamanick, B.: Prospective studies on the epidemiology of reproductive casualty: methods, findings and some implications, *Merrill Palmer Quarterly* 12 (1968) 27–43.

Knox, E.G. & Mahon, D.F.: Evaluation of infant at risk registers, *Archives of Disease in Childhood* 45 (1970) 634–639.

Reerink, J.D. et al.: Het project SMOCK. Opzet en enkele voorlopige resultaten, *Tijdschrift voor Jeugdgezondheidszorg* 21 (1989) 3–6.

Rutter, M., Tizard, J., Whitmore, K. (eds.): *Education, health and behaviour*, London 1970.

Rutter, M.: Epidemiological-longitudinal approaches to the study of development, in: Collins, W.A. (ed.): *The concept of development. The Minnesota Symposia on Child Psychology. Vol. 15*, Hillsdale (NJ) 1982.

Sameroff, A.J.: Transactional models in early social relations, *Human Development* 18 (1975) 65–79.

Sameroff, A.J. & Chandler, M.J.: Reproductive risk and the continuum of caretaking casualty, in: Horowitz, F.D. (ed.): *Review of child development research (Vol. 4)*, Chicago 1975.

Schlesinger-Was, E.A.: *Ontwikkelingsonderzoek voor zuigelingen en kleuters op het consultatiebureau*, Leiden 1981 (dissertation).

Werkgroep Van Wiechen: *Ontwikkelingsonderzoek op het consultatiebureau; werkboek bij het herziene Van Wiechenschema*, Zwolle: Kruisvereniging West-Overijssel, 1983.

Wilbrink-Griffioen, D. & Eyck, A.M. van: *Eindrapport: Evaluatie van het gebruik van het herziene Van Wiechenschema*, Leiden: Research voor Beleid, 1989.

Further reading

Anonymous: Developmental Screening (Editorial), *The Lancet* (1986) 1, 950–952.

Angulo-Laurent, M.S. & Schlesinger-Was, E.A.: Reactie van de Van Wiechen Werkgroep, *Tijdschrift voor Jeugdgezondheidszorg* 22 (1990) 6, 90–91.

Balledux, M., Mare, J. de, Winter, M. de: *Project Integrale Evaluatie Jeugdgezondheidszorg voor kinderen van 0–4 jaar. Literatuurstudies*, Utrecht: Rijksuniversiteit Utrecht, 1991.

Bos, M.W. & Winter, M. de (red.): *Jeugdgezondheidszorg in de toekomst*, Amsterdam 1989.

Canadian Task Force on the Periodic Health Examination: The periodic health examination. Task Force Report, *Canadian Medical Association Journal* 121 (1979) 1193–1254.

Chatab, J. & Kerkstra, A.: Gestandaardiseerde zorgverlening binnen de jeugd-gezondheidszorg voor 0–4 jarigen. Ideaal of werkelijkheid?, *Tijdschrift voor Sociale Gezondheidszorg* 69 (1991) 3, 61–68.

Cochrane, A.L. & Holland, W.W.: Validation of screening procedures, *British Medical Bulletin* 27 (1971) 3.

Collins, W.A. (ed.): *The concept of development. The Minnesota Symposia on Child Psychology. Vol. 15*, Hillsdale (NJ) 1982.

Drillien, C.M.: Developmental assessment and development screening, in: Drillien, C.M. & Drummond, M.B.: *Neurodevelopmental problems in early childhood*, London 1977.

Drillien, C.M. & Drummond, M.B.: *Neurodevelopmental problems in early childhood*, London 1977.

Dworkin, P.H.: British and American Recommendations for Developmental Monitoring: The Role of Surveillance, *Pediatrics* 84 (1989) 6, 1000–1010.

Foltz, A.: *An ounce of prevention. Child health politics under Medicaid*, Cambridge, Massachusetts 1982.

Frankenburg, W.K. & Camp, B.W. (eds.): *Pediatric screening tests*, Springfield (Ill) 1975.

Frankenburg, W.K., Chen, J., Thornton, S.M.: Common pitfalls in the evaluation of screening tests, *Journal of Pediatrics* 113 (1988) 1110–1113.

Gesell, A. & Amatruda, C.S.: Development diagnosis; normal and abnormal child development, in: Knobloch, H. & Pasamanick, B. (eds.): *Developmental diagnosis; the evaluation and management of normal and abnormal neuropsychologic development in infancy and early childhood*, Hagerstown: Harper & Row, 1974.

Glascoe, F.P., Martin, E.D., Humphrey, S.: Consumer reports. A Comparative Review of Developmental Screening Tests, *Pediatrics* 86 (1990) 4, 547–554.

Groenendaal, J., Rispens, J.: *Ontwikkeling en evaluatie van een signalerings-en begeleidingsmethodiek van psychosociale problemen en opvoedingsvragen t.b.v. de JGZ 0–4 jaar*, interne publikatie Project Integrale Evaluatie Jeugd-gezondheidszorg, Utrecht: Rijksuniversiteit Utrecht, 1991 (WP025).

Holt, K.S.: Screening for disease. Infancy and childhood, *The Lancet* November 2 (1974) 1057–1060.

Landelijke Commissie VTO: *Eerste rapport van de Landelijke Commissie VTO (ISG 3)*, Den Haag 1979.

Landelijke Commissie VTO: *Eindrapport van de Landelijke Commissie VTO (ISG 4)*, Den Haag 1981.

Macfarlane, A., Sefi, S., Cordeiro, M.: *Child Health, The Screening Tests*, New York 1989.

North, A.F.: Screening in child health care: where are we now and where are we going? *Pediatrics* 54 (1974) 631–640.

Pijning, H.F. & Swaveling-Pijning, M.: Consultatiebureau-arts en motorische ontwikkeling. Een ruimere interpretatie van het Van Wiechenschema, *Tijdschrift voor Jeugdgezondheidszorg* 22 (1990) 6, 86–90.

Ridder-Sluiter, J.G. de: *Vroegtijdige onderkenning van communicatieve ontwikkelingsstoornissen*, Meppel 1990 (dissertation).

Touwen, B.C.L.: Ontwikkelingsonderzoek en VTO-taal/spraak (inleiding), in: *Effectmaten voor de preventieve jeugdgezondheidszorg*, interne publikatie Project Integrale Evaluatie Jeugdgezondheidszorg, Utrecht: Rijkuniversiteit Utrecht, 1991 (WP022).

Vaandrager, G.J. (red.): *Ontwikkelingsonderzoek op het consultatiebureau voor zuigelingen en kleuters. Symposium ter gelegenheid van het afscheid van Betteke Schlesinger-Was*, Leiden 1987.

Wilson, J.M.G. & Jungner, G.: *Principles and practice of screening for disease (Public Health Papers no. 34)*, Genève: World Health Organization, 1968.

Winter, M. de: *Het voorspelbare kind. Vroegtijdige onderkenning van ontwikke-lingsstoornissen (VTO) in wetenschappelijk en sociaal-historisch perspectief*, Lisse 1986 (dissertation).

Winter, M. de: Vooren nadelen van gestandaardiseerd ontwikkelingsonderzoek op het consultatiebureau, in: Vaandrager, G.J. (red.): *Ontwikkelingsonderzoek op het consultatiebureau voor zuigelingen en kleuters. Symposium ter gelegenheid van het afscheid van Betteke Schlesinger-Was*, Leiden 1987.

Yankauer, A.: Child health supervision – is it worth it? (Commentaries), *Pediatrics* 52 (1973) 272–279.

7 Detection of speech and language disorders

Communicative development is linked with the cognitive, motor and socio-economic development of the child. These development fields influence one another. It is evident that disorders in communicative development can have considerable repercussions on the general development of young children.

In the last few years, Dutch Child Health Care for pre-school children has paid more and more attention to the detection of speech and language disorders. Until recently no specific method had been available for this purpose. The Van Wiechen[1] check-list (for psychomotor development) does indeed include a few speech and language items, but there proved to be a need for a standardized research instrument more specifically addressing linguistic and speech development (Schlesinger-Was 1986). With the aid and cooperation of the National Committee for the Early Detection of Developmental Disorders (Landelijke Commissie Vroegtijdige Onderkenning van Ontwikkelingsstoornissen) it was decided to construct a detection and surveillance test that would allow detection, within Child Health Care, of Dutch pre-school children with delayed and/or deviant linguistic development. The Early Detection test has two parts: there is a detection and information part targeting the communicative development of children between birth and 3 years of age (De Ridder-Sluiter 1990) and there is a surveillance part targeted at the language acquisition of children between the ages of 3–6 years (Gerritsen 1988).

Speech and language surveillance is a form of standardized programmed prevention, that is a systematic and standardized detection of disorders in the communicative development of all children from birth to 3 years of age. The surveillance may also serve a (more individual) counselling and support purpose: information about speech development and language acquisition can give parents an insight into the communicative development

---

[1]Partly based on the Denver Developmental Scale, the Van Wiechen check-list was developed in the early 1980s to promote the systematic examination of development (motor development, language and speech, personality and social behaviour) and to achieve uniform national registration. For details see Chapter 6, section 5.

of their child. In this way, parents can be helped in stimulating their child's communicative development. The following subjects are considered in this chapter: normal language acquisition and the disorders that may occur in it; the causes and consequences of such disorders; how to measure whether the aims set are reached. Then a number of methods are discussed, including the Early Detection language test. Finally the conclusions and the recommendations of the Project Group are reported.

7.1 Normal language acquisition

Normal speech development and language acquisition are characterized by great differences between individuals in both the speed and the pattern of development. This variation is explained by many medical, psychological and educational factors that influence the process of acquisition of speech and language. Two aspects of normal linguistic development are especially important for the detection of speech and language disorders: the period of sensitivity for language and the variation in speech and language acquisition. Most authors seem to agree that there is such a thing as a period of language sensitivity, during which language can be acquired most quickly and easily. After this period the learning process is much more laborious. It would be important for the detection of speech and language disorders to know how long this language sensitive period lasts, so that treatment can be started within this period. However, there seems to be no agreement on this point. Several authors mention periods as diverse as the first year and the seventh[2]. Eichenwald (1985) and some others do not believe there is any sensitive period at all.

7.2 Disorders in speech and language acquisition

Children who do not yet speak or do not speak well at the age at which they are expected to do so, are called language impaired (Goorhuis-Brouwer 1988). The question is when a child may be expected to start talking. Literature, both national and international, seems to lack consensus on this point. The ages mentioned vary between 9 and 18 months[3]. This would mean that language acquisition disorders may arise at

---

[2]Van der Lem & Baart de la Faille (1981), Kirkwood & Kirkwood (1983), Tervoort (1988), Goorhuis-Brouwer (1986).

[3]Griffith (1954), Gesell (1950), Schaerlaekens (1977), Menyuk (1977).

various moments, depending on the standard applied. An extra complication in this respect is that disorders or defects can also occur in the non-
verbal (pre-language) period. This implies, not only that the age at which a
child can be said to be language impaired is advanced, but also that the
term language acquisition disorders covers a very heterogeneous group of
disorders, relating to the course of non-verbal as well as verbal
communicative development.

There is a lack of clarity about the definition and description of language
acquisition disorders. Since various disciplines conduct research in this field
and each one employs its own terminology, it is difficult to compare
research from different disciplines. For this reason, the percentages for
prevalence that come up in various studies are markedly divergent: they
vary between 1% and 19.2% (MacKeith & Rutter 1972, Morley 1972,
Richman & Stevenson 1973, Snow 1977, Cantwell & Baker 1985,
Kalverboer 1985, Richman & Landsdown 1988, De Ridder-Sluiter 1990).
According to Rescorla (1989) prevalence decreases as the child grows older:
she finds a higher prevalence among 2-year-olds than among 3-year-olds.
This author ascribes the difference to a large number of late-developers[4].

7.3 Causes of disorders in language acquisition

Eight factors which may cause and/or influence disorders in linguistic
development can be deduced from the two major approaches to linguistic
development disorders: the psychomedical and the psycholinguistic
(Goorhuis-Brouwer 1988):

- hearing disorders
- abnormalities of the speech organs
- insufficient motor control of the speech organs
- brain damage in early childhood
- language offered by the environment
- cognition
- emotional development
- genetic factors.

---

[4]In a study by Rescorla (1989) it appeared that 50% of the children who were retarded in
speech behaviour at the age of 2 years 'had recovered spontaneously' at the age of 3 years.

Finally it should be remarked that mental retardation may also be the cause of such disorders.

7.4 Consequences of language acquisition disorders

The consequences of language acquisition disorders, as mentioned in international literature, can be classified in two groups: those affecting the child's behaviour and those affecting its learning achievement. There is consensus on the fact that language acquisition disorders may cause learning disorders and difficulties in reading and writing.[5] There is less unanimity on the effects on children's social behaviour. Writers including Rutter and Martin (1972) and Silva et al. (1983) are convinced that there is such a connection. Goorhuis-Brouwer (1988) however argues that in the literature, data on the relationship of language acquisition disorders and social behaviour are scarce. These disorders may also be the consequence of less than optimal living and development conditions. Moreover, in her opinion, other psychological and behavioural factors may be part determinants of the language problems.

7.5 Aim and outcome measurement of speech and language surveillance

As indicated in the introduction to this chapter, speech and language surveillance has two functions: detection (standardized programmed prevention) and support. To evaluate the detection function the following outcome measures may be considered:

- reduction of the number of infants/children suffering from linguistic development disorders
- fewer referrals to special schools because of communication disorders
- earlier diagnosis and treatment of speech and language problems.

---

[5]Aram and Nation (1980), Liebergott et al. (1984), Snijder (1984), Silva et al. (1983), Rutter (1972), Kalverboer (1985).

To evaluate the support function the following outcome measures may be drawn up:

- increase in parents' knowledge of linguistic and speech development

- fewer queries from parents with regard to their child's linguistic and speech development.

7.6 Methods for the detection of disorders in language acquisition

In this section the Early Detection language test developed in the Netherlands is discussed and compared with several other methods. These methods were selected because of their suitability for use at Child Health Clinics.

7.6.1 The Early Detection Language Project

At the instigation of the National Committee Early Detection (Landelijke Commissie VTO), the Early Detection language project was started in May 1981. Its aim was to design a detection and surveillance method with which to detect a retarded and/or deviant linguistic development in Dutch children between birth and 6 years of age. This project was carried out by the Netherlands Foundation for the Deaf and Hearing Impaired Child (Nederlandse Stichting voor het Dove en Slechthorende Kind NSDSK) and the Department for Developmental Psychology of Leiden University (RUL). The Foundation developed a detection test and an information instrument for children of 3 years or younger (Early Detection Language Project birth to 3 years) (De Ridder-Sluiter 1990); the RUL developed a surveillance test for 3–6 year olds (Early Detection language Project 3–6 years) (Gerritsen 1988).

7.6.1.1 Early Detection Language Project birth to 3 years

This surveillance method aims at the detection of children who have retarded and/or deviant communicative development and consists of two parts: a detection test and an information instrument (De Ridder-Sluiter 1990).

The detection test

The compilers of the test distinguish three major aspects in communicative development: productive (using language), receptive or comprehensive (understanding language) and interactive (with parents/environment). These three aspects are included in each phase of the test in the shape of questions put to parents or child. The choice of subjects and the timing of the test are chosen so as to ensure that 90% of the children will have a positive score (P90 age). The questions are put by a doctor or district nurse and are drawn up in a specific way, aimed not only at gaining insight into the 'yes' versus 'no' answer, but also at making it clearer to parents what the required communicative skills are. The preformulated way of putting questions also aims to increase the uniformity and reliability of testing. The test can be fitted into the regular practice of the clinic: it only takes a short time (about 2 minutes[6]), it is easy and unambiguous to handle and score and the timing coincides with the timing of visits to the clinic.

Although the test initially consisted of 10 sessions, the validity assessment showed that two or three successive sessions within a period of 6 months are sufficient to detect disorders or deviations. The validity was assessed by means of two follow-up surveys, 1 and 3 years after the use of the test[7]. Exact figures on validity and effectiveness of the method were not given, however. Users (clinical medical officers and district nurses) were also asked for their opinions. Generally they believe that the method can be fitted in well with the work in the clinic, that it is a useful supplement to this work and that it provides information on communicative development hitherto not available. Another positive side effect mentioned is that parents now pay more conscious attention to their child's communicative development. Finally, it should be noted that the Early Detection language test was designed for Dutch-speaking children. It does not seem possible, therefore, to detect disorders in the communicative development of children from an ethnic minority (whose mother tongue is not Dutch). The method was tried out in a number of test areas.

The information instrument

The information instrument was developed mainly to give parents insight into, and make them conscious of, the course of their child's communicative development as well as to increase the parents' ability to

---

[6]Research by De Ridder-Sluiter (1989) shows that after an initial period the test can be held in about 2 minutes.

[7]The follow-up survey included: the comprehension part of the Reynell Language Scales or, with children under 18 months, the mental scale of the Bayley Development Scale; analysis of a recording of the child's spontaneous use of language; two questionnaires for parents.

identify problems. At the moment the educational instrument is not yet used in pre-school Child Health Care; it is being used by way of trial in a number of courses for parents.

7.6.1.2 Early Detection Language Project 3–6 years

This method aims at the early detection of children with delayed and/or deviant language acquisition (Gerritsen 1988).

Theoretical considerations regarding linguistic development as well as practical demands for efficient and simple use have played their part in designing the surveillance method. The method can be used by clinics (pre-school children) as well as by Municipal Child Health Care (children between 4 and 6 years). According to the author, the test is always part of the Periodical Systematic Examination (PSE)[8]. The basic assumption is that no more than 10 minutes can be spent on testing and scoring. As is the case with the test for children up to 3 years old, this method is based on Bloom and Lahey's (1978) linguistic division in form, content and use.

The method is in three parts:

- The Language Surveillance Test (LST), the examination of the child, is the main element. There are three versions of the LST: for ages 3, 4 and 5 years. The LST is made up of items from tests on language, verbal intelligence and development currently in use in the Netherlands. It provides information on comprehension[9].

- The Parent Questionnaire (PQ) is in only one version for all three age groups. 'In compiling the Parents Questionnaire especially questions on linguistic development were selected which experts (see part 1 of Early Detection Language report 1982[10]) consider important to put to parents. In addition, the compilers drew on the stock of linguistic development questions that usually have to be answered by parents in language and development tests. These are especially concerned with the way in which the child enters into and keeps up communication and the extent to which it is capable

---

[8]The term 'PSE' is not normally used in Child Health Care literature. The author probably refers to Periodical Health Examination (PHE)

[9]As the author uses a number of different concepts it is not clear what is measured by LST. We cite Gerritsen 1988: 'The LST items mainly give an impression of the child's *knowledge* of the various language components...' (p. 24). 'The LST chiefly provides information on *comprehension*' (p. 188). 'The LST especially investigates *command of the language* at the relative age...' (p. 23).

[10]Ruiter, R. de: *Deelrapport 1 VTO-Taal (Part 1 Early Detection Language Report)*, Leiden University 1981.

of expressing itself fluently and clearly' (Gerritsen 1988)[11]. Most PQ questions are yes or no questions (with the exception of those aiming to record the child's speech acts). Questions are also included about background: on the parents' level of education, composition of the family, the father's and/or mother's employment and the reading habits in the family.

- The SQ (School Questionnaire) is also in one version and has been derived from the PQ.

'The three parts together provide a picture of the child's language performance in different situations, which is especially important in case of referral for further diagnostic examination and guidance' (Gerritsen 1988). The examination should be conducted at least twice between the ages of 3 and 6 years. With regard to reliability, validity and effectiveness of the method, the author puts forward the following arguments:

- The LST, PQ and SQ standards appear to be correct. However, they are not based on a representative national sample survey.

- The reliability of the LST is high for all ages. The SQ and PQ have a good internal consistency for all age groups, albeit that the consistency of SQ is better than that of PQ.

- LST, SQ and PQ validities appear to be good.

- As yet, nothing is known about the effectiveness of the programme.

The author also states that further testing (with large groups of children) is necessary for standardization, reliability and validity, and that research should be done into how far the tests can be used with 'foreign speakers'[12] as an indication of the measure in which the child is a 'Dutch speaker'.

The Early Detection language surveillance instrument for 3-year-olds is not used in pre-school Child Health Care. The version for 4- and 5-year-

---

[11]Here again the author is somewhat equivocal in the notions used. We cite Gerritsen 1988: 'The questions put to parents should therefore be targeted at the *perception of their child's general command* of the language, both with regard to *comprehension of spoken language and fluency*...The main thing is the extent to which and the way in which *the child is capable of carrying on a conversation*' (p. 24). 'The questionnaires for Parents (PQ) and School (SQ) give information on the level of *"conversation"* at home and at school' (p. 188). On page 121 it is stated that both the PQ and the SQ measure the *use of language.*

[12]Here the author alludes to children from an ethnic minority as well as to the use of 'regional language'.

olds is used, on a small scale, in both the pre-school Child Health Care and for the 4–19-year-olds. For instance, all 5-year-olds in the town of Enschede were screened using this instrument in the years 1990 and 1991. The final report, incorporating the results, was to be published in the autumn of 1992. The version for 5-year-olds is included in the speech therapy surveillance list published by the Nederlandse Vereniging voor Logopedie en Foniatrie (Dutch Association for Speech Therapy). In 1992, the method was used in Child Health Care in Flanders. Finally it should be noted that it is unclear in how far the two Early Detection language tests (for birth–3-year-olds and for 3–6-year-olds) link up and whether the results of the two methods are comparable.

7.6.2 The Language Development Survey

This method, evolved by Rescorla (1989), is a once-only surveillance method to be used for the entire population of children aged 2 years and is targeted at language use only. It is assumed that a child of that age has a vocabulary of at least 50 words and uses combinations of two or three words. This is checked by asking the parent(s) to fill in a questionnaire, which takes about 10 minutes. On the basis of the answers, a doctor can quickly assess speech development and language acquisition. According to the author's own research the reliability of the screening test varies between 0.86 and 0.99; there is also a high correlation with other tests (such as the Bayley Mental Development Scale, the Pre-School Language Scale and the Reynell Expressive and Receptive Language Scales); finally both the sensitivity (89%) and the specificity (86%) of the test are high.

7.6.3 Method of Bax, Hart and Jenkins (1980)

This method is intended for the whole population of children between 18 months and 4.5 years of age. There are four sessions during the period (18 months, 2 years, 3 years and 4.5 years). The authors emphasize that the assessment (by a paediatrician, a doctor or a health aide) must be made in an informal setting; in the first place because children are often rather uncooperative in a formal testing procedure, and secondly because they believe an informal procedure takes less time.

The content of the test is roughly as follows:

- 18 months: the number of words used by the child is counted; if the child is unwilling to talk the count is based on information from the parent(s)

- 2 years: the child is expected to use (many) more than 10 words and make two- or three-word combinations
- 3 years: the child should point to its nose, eyes and mouth; pictures are used to try and start a conversation with the child
- 4.5 years: the child is expected to use reasonably complex sentences in a conversation with the doctor.

The speech/language assessment should be part of the Periodic Health Examination (PHE) and the development examination. Data on validity and effectiveness are not available.

7.6.4 Minimum speech standards

These minimum speech standards were drawn up by Goorhuis-Brouwer (1986) as a help for '...general practitioners, paediatricians and other specialists, in general the people who are the first to be confronted with questions from worried parents...'. The minimum speech standards (six in the period 1–5 years of age) are minimum standards (with reference to the use of language) a child has to meet; if it falls short of these minimum standards, further assessment is desirable.

In short, the standards are:

- 1 year: much and varied prattling
- 1.5 years: speaks at least five words
- 2 years: speaks in two-word utterances
- 3 years: speaks in utterances of three to five words
- 4 years: speaks in plain and simple sentences, with a reasonably adjusted grammatical structure
- 5 years: speaks in reasonably well-formed sentences, including complex sentences.

There are no data on validity and effectiveness.

7.6.5 The use of parents' information

Many speech and language tests (including the Early Detection language test) use information from parents. Parents were given such an important role on the one hand out of necessity: very young children in particular are not easily inclined to talk to strange people in a strange situation; on the other hand many authors[13] are of the opinion that parents are the most suitable and most expert informants as far as their child's speech and linguistic development is concerned. The measure of reliability of parental information is a generally recognized problem. Attempts are made to overcome this drawback by structuring questionnaires and interviews so as to ensure that the information is as reliable as possible. A number of authors[14] hold that the problem cannot be solved by well-structured questionnaires and interviews; they believe that parents can supply reliable information only on the child's use of language and not about its comprehension, because parents often (wrongly) take for granted that their child understands all they say.

7.6.6 Comparing the various methods

A comparison of the above methods shows there to be considerable differences between the tests as far as the ages are concerned at which they are used for the first time. Apparently there is no consensus about the age at which the detection of disorders or deviations can or should be started; normal communicative development is characterized by large variations in pace and pattern; the distinction between late developers and those whose are language impaired is hard to make: identification at an early age yields many false positives; but later on (when late developer is out of the question) may easily be too late to intervene successfully. Comparison also shows that there is no consensus on the question whether disorders in linguistic development can be detected by a once-only test (such as Rescorla's) or whether a longitudinal method (such as the Early Detection language test) is needed. The compilers of the Early Detection language test for children from birth to 3 years believe that a number of shorter sessions across a longer span of time will produce a more reliable assessment of the course of communicative development than a once-only session. Moreover, such longitudinal examining takes into account, so they say, the spread in the course of communicative development (De Ridder-Sluiter & Van der Lem 1988). Finally, there appears to be no consensus on the question of what could or should be the minimum examination frequency in order to allow the detection of disorders. In the methods described above different frequencies are used.

---

[13]Including De Ridder-Sluiter (1989), Bates et al. (1979, 1983), Dale et al. (1989), Rescorla (1989), Benedict (1979).

[14]Including Rescorla (1989), Goorhuis-Brouwer (1986).

7.7 The importance of an adequate follow-up route

As indicated in section 7.3 the causes of communication disorders may be very diverse. Therefore it is extremely important that after identification the follow-up route is of a multidisciplinary nature. De Ridder-Sluiter (1989) arrives at the conclusion that: 'Diagnosing children with delayed and/or deviant communicative development requires expertise and a multidisciplinary approach, in which various developmental aspects have to be examined...The care that follows may consist of speech/language therapy, but may also be in the medical and/or psychological/educational fields'.

7.8 Conclusions

With the development of the Early Detection language test another step was taken in the standardization of the detection of developmental disorders in young children. Although the Early Detection language test for birth to 3-year-olds has proved to be an adequate test for detection, the follow-up route after identification (diagnosis and treatment) is still insufficiently known. The Early Detection language test is being put into use in a number of trial areas.

7.9 Recommendations

- At the request of the Project Group the collection of data from the implementation study has been adapted to the cost-effectiveness model of Erasmus University. When carrying out this cost-effectiveness analysis it is recommended that particular attention be paid to the follow-up route after the detection of the disorder.

- It is recommended that national implementation of the Early Detection language test be proceeded with only if it appears from the implementation study mentioned in the first recommendation that the test produces sufficient effect at acceptable cost.

References

Aram, D.M. & Nation, J.E.: Preschool language disorders and subsequent language academic difficulties, *Journal of Communication Disorders* 13 (1980) 150–159.

Bates, E., Benigni, L., Bretherton, J., Camaioni, L., Volterra, V.: From gesture to first word: on cognitive and social prerequisites, in: Lewis, M. & Rosenblum, L. (eds.): *Interaction, conversation and the development of language*, New York: John Wiley & Sons, 1979.

Bates, E., Bretherton, I, Shore, C., McKnew, S.: Names, gestures and objects: symbolization in infancy and aphasia, in: Nelson, K. (ed.): *Children's language (Vol. 4)*, Hillsdale, NJ: Lawrence Erlbaum, 1983.

Bax, M., Hart, H., Jenkins, S.: Assessment of speech and language development in the young child, *Pediatrics* 66 (1980) 350–354.

Benedict, H.: Early lexical development: comprehension and production, *Journal of Child Language* 6 (1979) 183–201.

Bloom, L. & Lahey, M.: *Language development and language disorders*, New York: John Wiley & Sons, 1978.

Cantwell, C.P. & Baker, L.: Psychiatric disorders in children with speech and language retardation: a critical review, *Archives of General Psychiatry* 34 (1985) 583–589.

Dale, Ph.S., Bates, E., Reznick, J.S., Morisset, C.: The validity of a parent report instrument of child language at twenty months, *Journal of Child Language* 16 (1989) 239–249.

Eichenwald, H.: Developments in diagnosing and treating otitis media, *American Family Physician* 31 (1985) 155–164.

Gesell, A.: *The first five years of life*, London: Methuen & Co. Ltd., 1950.

Gerritsen, F.M.E.: *VTO taalscreening 3- tot 6-jarigen; de ontwikkeling van een taalscreeningsinstrumentarium voor gebruik in de jeugdgezondheidszorg*, Amsterdam/Lisse 1988 (dissertation).

Goorhuis-Brouwer, S.M.: Spraaken taalontwikkelingsstoornissen. Verwijzings- criteria, diagnostiek en mogelijkheden tot behandeling, *Modern Medicine* January (1986) 143–146.

Goorhuis-Brouwer, S.M.: *Gesprekspartners? Taalontwikkelings-stoornissen als pedagogisch probleem, een verkenning*, Amersfoort/Leuven: ACCO, 1988 (dissertation).

Griffith, R.: *The abilities of babies*, London: University of London Press, 1954.

Kalverboer, A.F.: Over de vroegtijdige onderkenning van dyslexie, in: Ley, A.M. van der & Stevens, L.M. (red.): *Dyslexie*, Lisse: Swets & Zeitlinger, 1985.

Kirkwood, C.R. & Kirkwood, M.E.: Otitis media and learning disabilities; the case for a causal relationship, *Journal of Family Practitioner* 17 (1983) 219–227.

Lem, G.J. van der & Baart de la Faille, L.: Vroegtijdige opsporing van gehoorstoornissen, *Nederlands Tijdschrift voor Geneeskunde* 51 (1981) 2104–2109.

Liebergott, H.J.W., Bashir, A.S, Schultz, M.C.: Dancing around and making strange noises, in: Holland, A. (ed.): *Language disorders in children*, San Diego: College Hill Press, 1984.

MacKeith, R.C. & Rutter, M.: A note on the prevalence of speech and language disorders, in: Rutter, M. & Martin, J.A.M. (eds.): *The child with delayed speech*, London: William Heinemann Medical Books Ltd., 1972.

Menyuk, P.: *Kind en taalontwikkeling*, Utrecht: Spectrum, 1977.

Morley, M.E.: *The development and disorders of speech in childhood*, Edinburgh: Churchill Livingstone, 1972.

Rescorla, L: The Language Development Survey: a screening tool for delayed language in toddlers, *Journal of Speech and Hearing Disorders* 54 (1989) 587–599.

Richman, N. & Landsdown, R.: *Problems of preschool children*, New York: John Wiley & Sons, 1988.

Richman, N. & Stevenson, J.: Language delay in 3 years olds. Family and social factors, *Acta Paedakto Belgica* 30 (1973) 213–219.

Ridder-Sluiter, J.G. & Lem, G.J. van der: Project VTO-taal biedt instrumenten voor signalering en voorlichting, *Maatschappelijke Gezondheidszorg* 16 (1988) 28–31.

Ridder-Sluiter, J.G. de: *Vroegtijdige onderkenning van communicatieve ontwikkelingsstoornissen*, Meppel 1990 (dissertation).

Rutter, M. & Martin, J.A.M.: *The child with delayed speech*, London: William Heinemann Medical Books Ltd., 1972.

Schaerlaekens, A.M.: *De taalontwikkeling van het kind. Een oriëntatie in het Nederlandstalig onderzoek*, Groningen: Wolters Noordhof, 1977.

Schlesinger-Was, E.A.: *Vroege opsporing van gehoorstoornissen in het kader van de jeugdgezondheidszorg voor zuigelingen en kleuters*, Leiden: NIPG/TNO, 1986.

Silva, P.A., McGee, R., Williams, S.M.: Developmental language delay from three to seven years and its significance for low intelligence and reading difficulties at age seven, *Developmental Medicine and Child Neurology* 25 (1983) 783–793.

Snijder, L.: Developmental language disorders: elementary school age, in: Holland, A. (ed.): *Language disorders in children*, San Diego: College Hill Press, 1984.

Snow, C.E.: The development of conversation between mothers and babies, *Child Language* 4 (1977) 1–22.

Further reading

Balledux, M., Mare, J. de, Winter, M. de: *Project Integrale Evaluatie Jeugd-gezondheidszorg voor kinderen van 0–4 jaar. Literatuurstudies*, Utrecht: Rijksuniversiteit Utrecht, 1991.

Bishop, D.V.M., Edmundson, A.: Language impaired 4-year-olds: distinguishing transient from persistent impairment, *Journal of Speech and Hearing Disorders* 52 (1987) 156–173.

Bzoch, K.R. & League, R.: *Assessing language skills in infancy*, Baltimore: University Park Press, 1971.

Groen, Th. & Bosman, E.: Screening op ontwikkelingsstoornissen van spraak, taal en stem, *Logopedie en Foniatrie* 61 (1989) 136–138.

Haber, J.S & Norris, M.: The Texas Preschool Screening Inventory. A simple screening device for language and learning disorders, in: Frankenburg, W.K., Emde, R.N., Sullivan, J.W.: *Early identification of children at risk. An international perspective*, New York/London: Plenum Press, 1985.

Hixon, Th.J., Shriberg, L.D., Saxman, J.H. (eds.): *Introduction to communication disorders*, Englewood Cliffs: Prentice-Hall, 1980.

Holland, A.L. (ed.): *Language disorders in children*, San Diego: College Hill Press, 1984.

Ierland, M.S. van: Onderkenning en opvang van kinderen met taalontwikkelingsstoornissen: enkele knelpunten, *Logopedie en Foniatrie* 54 (1982) 91–103.

Martin, J.A.M.: *Voice, speech, and the language in the child: development and disorder*, Wenen: Springer-Verlag, 1981.

Meulen, Sj. van der, Doets, B., Metz, N.G. (red.): *Taalontwikkelingsstoornissen: onderzoek en behandeling*, Lisse: Swets & Zeitlinger, 1985.

Ridder-Sluiter, J.G. de: *Eindverslag projekt VTO-taal 0–3 jaar. Vroegtijdige onderkenning van een vertraagde en/of afwijkende communicatieve ontwikkeling bij kinderen van 0-3 jaar*, Amsterdam: NSDSK, 1989.

Ruiter, R. de: *Deelrapport 1 VTO-Taal*, Leiden: Rijksuniversiteit Leiden, 1981.

Stevenson, J.: Predictive value of speech and language screening, *Developmental Medicine and Child Neurology* 26 (1984) 528–538.

Tervoort, B.T.: Taalontwikkeling en taalontwikkelingsstoornissen; een overzicht in vogelvlucht, *Logopedie en Foniatrie* 60 (1988) 70–76.

Touwen, B.C.L.: Ontwikkelingsonderzoek en VTO-taal/spraak (inleiding), in: *Effectmaten voor de preventieve jeugdgezondheidszorg* (WP022), interne publikatie Project Integrale Evaluatie Jeugdgezondheidszorg, Utrecht: Rijkuniversiteit Utrecht, 1991.

8 The periodic health examination

The general objective of pre-school Child Health Care as described in Chapter 1, is to promote, monitor and secure the healthy physical, mental and social development of young children. For years, an objective of this kind has been realized through sessions at clinics, home visits and health education groups. Chapter 8 primarily concerns individual sessions in child health clinics. In the day-to-day practice of clinics in the Netherlands, various methods of prevention are used. These are integrated in a single coordinated procedure: the giving of check ups, health education and advice by the doctor and/or nurse at regular intervals, on the basis of a fixed notification schedule. Until now, this was referred to as the periodic medical examination. The definition and description of the periodic medical examination involves numerous problems. Taken literally, periodic medical examination means regular (periodic) examination by a doctor (medical examination). Obviously, this description as it stands is not satisfactory; it conveys no more than that a certain official regularly does something on the basis of his or her professional background. What this official does, and how often he or she does it, appears to be flexible: time and time again, the content and procedures of the periodic medical examination have been adapted to changing insights, not only in the course of the history of pre-school Child Health Care, but also today there are enormous differences internationally. In the Netherlands, for example, the term periodic medical examination has come to refer to the longitudinal follow-up and assessment of the growth and development of the young child including, of course, history taking and the giving of advice as needed. Depending on the definition that is chosen, the periodic medical examination is taken to mean either the regular physical examination alone, or a combination of the physical examination, screenings, developmental assessment, educational prevention activities and counselling, health education, and sometimes also immunization. A broad definition of this kind is similar to what is referred to in the English-speaking world as Child Health Surveillance.[1] In the United

---

[1]Hall (1989) describes Child Health Surveillance as 'a set of activities which are initiated by professionals. It includes the oversight of the physical, social and emotional health and development of all children; measurement and recording of physical growth; monitoring of developmental progress; offering and arranging intervention when necessary; prevention of disease by immunization and other means; and health education'.

Kingdom, a working party recently proposed that the periodic health examination within the framework of Child Health Care be basically restricted to a number of 'proven' effective screening and health education methods. In addition to this, parents are to be asked whether they have any problems with respect to other health aspects. In this way, the initiative for further examination, assessment and advice is left partly to the parents (Hall 1989). This procedure would drastically reduce the frequency with which the Child Health Clinics in the United Kingdom send out notifications, and at the same time would create the option of 'open clinics'[2].

For various reasons, the term periodic medical examination is no longer adequate. Firstly, the methods available for health assessment have become highly differentiated over the past decades. In various domains in the field of health and development, specific research methods, often standardized, have been developed which now operate more or less independently within the structure of the clinics. In chronological order, the most striking examples of these are the hearing test (Ewing method), developmental assessment (Van Wiechen check-list[3]), examination of the eyes (Early Detection vision) and the language/speech test (Early Detection language). Secondly, the term medical puts too much emphasis on somatic aspects. Although physical health is a decisive factor in the overall wellbeing of the child, its psychosocial development, its upbringing and social background are also important factors and are given a lot of attention in pre-school Child Health Care. In this connection, De Jonge (1992) points out that the term medical is somewhat inappropriate, precisely because of its curative connotation. In most cases, the children who are being examined are healthy and do not require a cure[4].

Thirdly, the work of the clinics is traditionally multidisciplinary: for many years now, the process of promoting, monitoring and securing the health and welfare of the child and its parents, has involved both doctors and nurses, assisted in recent years by nutritionists and educational

---

[2]The British programme that is discussed here has been implemented in a limited number of regions in the United Kingdom. There is no question as yet of implementation at the national level. At present, the programme is being tried and evaluated in the pilot region of Oxfordshire and in several others.

[3]Partly based on the Denver Developmental Scale, the Van Wiechen check-list was developed in the early 1980s to promote the systematic examination of development (motor development, language and speech, personality and social behaviour) and to achieve uniform national registration. For details see Chapter 6 section 5.

[4]In an editorial in the *Tijdschrift voor Jeugdgezondheidszorg* (Child Health Care Gazette), De Jonge proposes that the term periodic medical examination be replaced by periodic health contact. According to the author, the term examination is not correct either because it does not convey the interactive aspect.

specialists[5]. Nurses prove to fulfil an important role as observers of the combined mental and physical aspects of health.

As a result of these developments, the term periodic medical examination no longer fills the bill. It wrongly suggests a kind of methodological and disciplinary uniformity, while the practical situation that has developed is actually one of diversity. However, because the concept of periodic medical examination has been generally adopted by professionals, there have been many attempts to give the old term a new meaning. An unwelcome result of this is that quite a few, often contradictory, definitions of periodic medical examination are used, varying from very narrow definitions (the aggregate of scientifically recognized screening methods), to very broad definitions (the integral assessment and promotion of health and welfare).

The Project Group that was assigned the integral evaluation of Dutch pre-school Child Health Care devoted many discussions to this definition issue. These discussions have encompassed the whole topic of pre-school Child Health Care. Indeed, proponents of the broad definition think of the examination as a periodic health examination, which is nothing more, nor less, than the totality of the activities that are carried out by clinics in the Netherlands. The integral promotion and assessment of the health and welfare of the child and its parents includes history taking, physical and psychosocial examination, the drawing up of a health profile, health education, and counselling. Proponents of a narrow definition (as reflected, for example, in the British model put forward by Hall and others, which is discussed in detail below) tend to hold the view that a programme for periodic health examination that is actively offered to parents should include only screenings that have been proved reliable and valid.

Within the framework of the Project on the Integral Evaluation of Child Health Care (Project Integrale Evaluatie Jeugdgezondheidszorg) it was decided that as many elements of pre-school Child Health Care as possible would be assessed separately. This procedure has resulted, among other things, in separate studies on the standardized methods of prevention that are common in the clinics and which, according to some, constitute an integral part of the periodic health examination. According to others, they should be assessed independently (see the foregoing chapters). The conclusion that the term periodic medical examination obscures rather than clarifies, seems justified. The concept of a periodic medical examination, which may formerly have served a purpose, today appears to obstruct clear thinking about the desirable content of modern pre-school Child Health Care. For all these reasons, we use the term periodic health

---

[5]The appointment of nutritionists and educational experts depends on the policy of the regional Community Health Care organization in question.

examination here in its broadest sense, which we define as follows: the periodic health examination in pre-school Child Health Care is a system of longitudinal observation and counselling, aimed at monitoring and supervising growth and development, at promoting health, as well as at the identification of diseases, disorders or health-threatening factors. It includes history-taking, preventive physical and psychosocial examination, screening, health education, giving advice, counselling and, if necessary, referral.

Data obtained by means of the periodic health examination can, and should, fulfil an important role in establishing data relating to incidence and prevalence for epidemiological research.

However, from the point of view of evaluating the outcome, it is clear that there is no way to avoid a functional subdivision of this definition. As stated above, it was decided that a number of clearly defined methods would be assessed separately in the evaluation study. A number of specific standardized components have already been addressed in the foregoing chapters. Standardized components concerning upbringing and health education are considered in subsequent chapters. In this chapter, we deal specifically with the various elements of the periodic health examination. Subsequently, the most important similarities and differences between the Dutch and British systems of periodic health examination are looked at, with the idea of listing the advantages and disadvantages of each. This particularly concerns the degree of standardization and the related degree of structuring (frequent appointments versus a limited appointment schedule with open clinics).

8.1 The periodic health examination: history taking, examination and interview

In the Netherlands, the periodic health examination session takes approximately 10 minutes on average. It will be obvious that not all the aspects of the periodic health examination mentioned below can be dealt with in each session.

8.1.1 History taking

History taking involves the gathering of information about the period prior to the session. The parents are asked whether there is anything that they are concerned about or whether they have any questions. This is followed by functional assessment geared to the age of the child concerned. Questions are asked about aspects of care, safety and family life. With the help of this information, a health profile of the child can be drawn up (Dutch Association for Child Health Care; Nederlandse Vereniging voor Jeugdgezondheidszorg NVJG 1990). To do this, indicators for the state of health can be used as a guideline. The Dutch Association for Child Health Care (NVJG) lists the following: 'composition of the family (mother/mother role, father/father role, children, other members of the household), hereditary defects (a dozen diseases and deviations), history (illnesses, accidents, traumatic events, vaccinations), appearance (general impression, skin, neck, trunk, extremities, genitalia), growth (height and weight), development (motor, mental, including language skills and speech), and vital functions (sleeping, playing, eating/excretion, sensorimotor functions, control of bodily functions, independence, autonomic reactions' (NVJG 1990).

8.1.2 The examination

Both socio-medical and nursing consultations can include many kinds of tests. Moreover, a distinction can be made between standardized prevention measures and prevention to measure. Standardized prevention measures are formalized prevention programmes that are actively offered to all children at fixed moments (that is, without there being any question of a request for help). Prevention to measure concerns matters that are raised during the contact with the health worker, or on the initiative of the health worker on the basis of his findings and his knowledge of individual health risks, or at the request of the client.[6,7] Standardized and individualized

---

[6]The category examination requested occurs regularly during sessions, for example, with respect to so-called minor ailments. These are external 'defects' that can be observed in an infant, which the parents do not know the seriousness of. Examples of such minor ailments are: cutis marmorata, haemangioma cavernosum, nappy rash, mastitis neonatorum, milia, mongolian spot, congenital umbilical hernia, tightness of the foreskin, seborrheic eczema (cradle cap), and stasis of (purulent) lacrimal fluid in the corner of the eye during the first month of life (Van Wieringen 1991, personal communication).

[7]In addition to standardized screenings, Butler distinguishes two other components of individual Child Health Surveillance namely, case-finding (also called opportunistic screening) and non-specific oversight. He describes the latter component as 'the vigilant supervision of all aspects of the health and wellbeing of children whenever they come into contact with health care professionals'. It is concerned with 'seeing whether anything is wrong' rather than with 'looking for a particular condition'. However, with respect to this surveillance component, Butler draws attention to an important evaluation problem: whatever the importance of this form of 'many-faceted diagnostic awareness' might be, it is virtually impossible to quantify or measure. 'How much of this kind of oversight is done, by whom, at what cost, and to what effect, are questions upon which the literature can throw almost no light' (Butler 1989).

forms of prevention merge during sessions in Child Health Care. Strictly speaking, the first form of examination is basic health care (ideally, a package of research activities, based on epidemiological data, that is actively offered to all members of the target group in the absence of complaints and/or a request for help), and the second is primary health care, namely, diagnostic tests indicated by specific problems/complaints (Burgmeijer et al. 1991).

In addition to the observation of the child, and of the interaction between the child and its parents, the child may be examined for various aspects of health: physical health, growth and development (including biometric tests, examination of the eyes, ear-nose-throat, digestive system, heart and blood vessels, urogenital tract, locomotor and skin), psycho-motor development and examination of language and speech development. Apart from the standardized components (such as screenings, the Van Wiechen check-list, Early Detection vision and suchlike), there appears to be little consistency regarding which aspects are examined in each individual child, either in the Netherlands (Chatab 1989) or internation-ally. Section 8.2 deals with proposals for further formalization of the periodic health examination.

8.1.3 The interview

Each session is concluded with an interview in which, on the basis of the findings of the history and the physical examination, the health, growth and development of the child are discussed with the parents. This interview can cover various topics, the parents may be given advice and information (geared to the individual situation of the child and the parent, but also about general matters that are relevant for all children and their parents. These are matters concerning vaccinations, development, upbringing, care, nutrition and safety); also, parents who are concerned about their child can be reassured. With other parents the suspicion that there is a disorder may be discussed, or the parent-child relationship, problems of upbringing and so on.

8.2 Towards further formalization of the periodic health examination in the Netherlands

In recent years, the groups of professionals involved in pre-school Child Health Care have striven for further standardization of components of the periodic health examination. An appropriate method is protocol development, a procedure that is used in medical research in primary and secondary health care (Vissers 1983), and also in respect to health education for patients (Cuisinier & Jonkers 1986). A protocol is defined as 'the operational reflection of the information that is available at any given time' (Vissers, 1983), and constitutes the explicit formulation of a procedure based on scientific consensus that can serve as a guideline and as an instrument for evaluating professional action. With respect to the periodic health examination, a Working Party consisting of former Provincial Child Health Care Officers (Provinciaal Artsen Jeugdgezondheidszorg) recently published a report that can be regarded as a first step towards formalization (Burgmeijer et al. 1991). The aim of the study was to provide a sound basis for the work of doctors in clinics. In his foreword, Vaandrager states 'this manual for periodic health examination in clinics can be regarded as a first step on the way to a protocol'. The authors hope that, with the publication of this manual, the variations in what is examined in individual children, as well as the different ways of carrying out the examinations will be reduced on the basis of the conviction that 'insight and self-confidence of both the clinical team and the parents can be increased by standardization of the follow-up of the child's development' (Burgmeijer et al. 1991). In the manual, the working definition of periodic health examination used by the Working Party is: patient history and physical examination. A number of components of the periodic health examination found in the outline of the programme have not been included in the study itself because detailed descriptions of these are already available. Examples are: auditory screening, testing on the basis of the Van Wiechen check-list, implementation of the Early Detection method, and immunization.

With regard to the aims of the periodic health examination, the manual states: 'periodic health examination enables the doctor in the clinic to assess the state of health of children who visit the clinic at fixed times'. Two questions need to be answered: does the child have any disorders/defects? and – the question that parents ask – 'Is my child healthy, and if so, is he/she as healthy as possible?'

The programme recommended in the periodic health examination manual is based on a combination of available epidemiological data and professional consensus. In drawing up the programme, a large number of medical specialists were consulted. As shown in the scheme below, the recommended programme consists of 16 sessions[8] in the clinic:

---

[8]The authors point out that the 16 health clinic sessions can be reduced to 14 by combining the tests for 5 and 6 months at 6 months, and by combining those for 7 and 9 months at 8 months.

N.B. The tests marked with an asterisk (*) can also be carried out by the district nurse. The role of the district nurse is not included in this programme except where it concerns medical action.

6–8 days		PKU/CHT screening*
1 month	biometry	weight*
		circumference of the head*
		crown–heel length*
	psychomotor development	exploratory neuro-developmental assessment
		Van Wiechen check-list
	eyes	inspection
		eye movements
		pupillary reflex
		refraction of light
	ear-nose-throat	inspection of the mouth, throat, nose, ears, neck
		palpation of cervical region
	digestive system	nutritional state
		fluid balance
		inspection of the mouth
		inspection, auscultation and palpation of the abdomen
	heart, blood vessels	general inspection
		inspection and palpation of the thorax
		auscultation of the heart
		palpation/percussion of liver
		palpation femoral artery
	urogenital tract	inspection external genitalia
		inspection/palpation testes
	locomotor	scoliosiometry
		check for CDH
		alignment knee joint (knock knees, bow-legs)
		check for deformities of the foot
	skin	inspection

2 months	biometry	weight[*] circumference of the head[*]
	psycho-motor development	Van Wiechen check-list
	eyes	inspection
	digestive system	nutritional state fluid balance inspection mouth/teeth inspection, auscultation and palpation of the abdomen
	heart, blood vessels	general inspection inspection and palpation of the thorax auscultation of the heart palpation/percussion of liver palpation femoral artery
	skin	inspection
3 months	biometry	crown–heel length[*] weight[*] circumference of the head[*]
	psycho-motor development	Van Wiechen check-list
	eyes	inspection
	digestive system	nutritional state fluid balance inspection mouth/teeth inspection, auscultation and palpation of the abdomen
	heart, blood vessels	general inspection inspection and palpation of the thorax auscultation of the heart palpation/percussion of liver palpation femoral artery
	locomotor	scoliosiometry check for deformities of the foot
	skin	inspection
	immunization	DPT/polio-1[*]

4 months	biometry	weight[*] circumference of the head[*]
	immunization	DPT/polio-2[*]
5 months	biometry	weight[*] circumference of the head[*]
	immunization	DPT/polio-3[*]
	locomotor	check for CDH
6 months	biometry	crown–heel length[*] weight[*] circumference of the head[*]
	psycho-motor	Van Wiechen check-list[9]
	digestive system	nutritional state fluid balance inspection mouth/teeth inspection, auscultation and palpation of the abdomen
	heart, blood vessels	general inspection inspection and palpation of the thorax auscultation of the heart palpation/percussion of liver palpation femoral artery
	locomotor	scoliosiometry check for CDH alignment knee joint (knock knees, bow-legs) check for deformities foot
	skin	inspection
7 months	eyes	Eearly Detection method
9 months	biometry	crown–heel length[*] weight[*] circumference of the head[*]
	psycho-motor development	Van Wiechen check-list

---

[9]In the outline of the programme in the book by Burgmeijer et al (1991), the administering of the Van Wiechen check-list at 6 months was erroneously omitted.

	ear-nose-throat	Ewing auditory screening or CAPAS (Compact Amsterdam Pedo-Audiometric Screener)*
	digestive system	nutritional state fluid balance inspection mouth/teeth inspection, auscultation and palpation of the abdomen
	locomotor	scoliosiometry
	skin	inspection
11–12 months	biometry	crown–heel length* weight* circumference of the head*
	immunization	DPT/polio-4*
	psycho-motor development	Van Wiechen check-list
	digestive system	nutritional state fluid balance inspection mouth/teeth inspection, auscultation and palpation of the abdomen
	locomotor	scoliosiometry check for CDH check for foot deformities
	skin	inspection
14 months	biometry immunization	weight* MMR-1*
15 months	psycho-motor development	Van Wiechen check-list*
18 months	biometry	height* weight*
	psycho-motor development	Van Wiechen check-list
	eyes	Early Detection method
	locomotor	scoliosiometry alignment knee joint (knock knees, bow-legs) check for foot deformities

24 months	biometry	height[*] weight[*]
	psycho-motor development	Van Wiechen check-list[*]
	digestive system	nutritional state inspection mouth/teeth inspection, auscultation and palpation of the abdomen
	heart, blood vessels	general inspection inspection and palpation of the thorax auscultation of the heart palpation/percussion of liver
	locomotor	scoliosiometry alignment knee joint (knock knees, bow-legs) check for foot deformities
	skin	inspection
30 months	psycho-motor development	Van Wiechen check-list[*]
36 months	biometry	height[*] weight[*]
	psycho-moto development	Van Wiechen check-list[*]
	digestive system	nutritional state inspection mouth/teeth inspection, auscultation and palpation of the abdomen
	heart, blood vessels	general inspection inspection and palpation of the thorax auscultation of the heart palpation/percussion of liver
	locomotor	scoliosiometry alignment knee joint (knock knees, bow-legs) check for foot deformities
	skin	inspection

45–48 months	biometry	height[*] weight[*]
	psycho-motor development	Van Wiechen check-list[*]
	eyes	Early Detection method test visual acuity[*]
	digestive system	nutritional state inspection mouth/teeth inspection, auscultation and palpation of the abdomen
	heart, blood vessels	general inspection inspection and palpation of the thorax auscultation of the heart palpation/percussion of liver
	locomotor	scoliosiometry alignment knee joint (knock knees, bow-legs) check for foot deformities
	skin	inspection
	immunization	DT/polio-5[*]

A more detailed version of this scheme, in Dutch, is given in: Burgmeijer, R.J.F., Boeken Kruger-Mangunkusumo, R.S. Fernandes, J. (ed.): *Periodiek Geneeskundig Onderzoek: een praktijkboek voor de jeugdgezondheidszorg*, Utrecht, 1991.

Within the framework of the Project Integral Evaluation of Child Health Care (Project Integrale Evaluatie) there was no opportunity to look at the programme proposed by this Working Party from the point of view of effectiveness. However, it should be stated that the fact that such a protocol becomes available constitutes an important prerequisite and is absolutely indispensable for carrying out an empirical study on the effectiveness of the periodic health examination. Experts in the Project Group have drawn up a large number of outcome measures that can be used in a possible evaluation of the effectiveness of this programme. In the opinion of the Project Group the initiation of such an effectiveness study in one or more trial regions is strongly advisable. If such a study should show that the proposed periodic health examination programme is effective and efficient, this would have important consequences in practice: at the moment, a less frequent notification schedule is used in many parts of the Netherlands, while the present length of time for each child is inadequate to carry out the proposed programme in full.

8.3 The British Joint Working Party on Child Health Surveillance

A survey of the content, frequency and implementation of sessions held within the framework of Child Health Surveillance in 138 of the 193 Health Districts in the United Kingdom in 1981, prompted the founding of the British Joint Working Party on Child Health Surveillance in 1986. From this study it appeared that there were substantial differences between the Districts, not only with respect to content, but also the number of sessions per child, and the person who performed them (Macfarlane & Pillay 1984). Further analysis has shown that the differences between the Districts were not related to differences between the populations receiving care[10]. The authors query the reasons for the different programmes and the factors on which the different programmes were based. They take the view that it ought to be possible to come to an agreement about the content of a Child Health Surveillance Programme at a national level: 'We would therefore suggest that all those concerned...should meet and jointly agree on a national policy of child health surveillance, based on such evidence as is available at the moment, and that such a policy should be continuously evaluated' (Macfarlane & Pillay 1984).

This idea was realized in 1986 with the founding of a national Working Party whose task was 'to review and comment on current practice in child health surveillance in the United Kingdom and to make recommendations for future practice' (Hall 1989). The Working Party consisted of representatives from the major (para)medical organizations that are involved in the implementation of Child Health Surveillance[11]. After two years, the Working Party drew up a draft report. This draft report was sent for comment to all organizations that have vested interests in the health of young children, before the Working Party officially published its

---

[10]Differences with respect to urbanization, the percentage of immigrants, the percentage of unemployed persons, lower social classes, and suchlike.

[11]The British Paediatric Association, the Royal College of General Practitioners, the General Medical Services Committee of the British Medical Association, the Health Visitors Association, and the Royal College of Nursing.

recommendations (Hall 1989). The aim of the Working Party was to study the value of the existing surveillance programmes in the light of the results of current scientific research. It was intended to recommend a new national programme that, with respect to content and frequency, would be based on scientific data.

Two important questions were left aside. First of all, the question of who can best carry out Child Health Care (the general practitioner, the clinical medical officer, or the child health visitor[12]). The British Working Party deliberately wished to keep this issue out of the discussion on content to avoid confusion of political and scientific arguments. Consequently, the Working Party did not take a decision on this question. Another point that was kept out of the study by the Working Party was the whole area of primary prevention (immunization, health promotion, and parent counselling). The work of the British Working Party focused on the early detection of diseases, defects and disorders (secondary prevention). In the report, the observation is made that, although both matters (primary and secondary prevention) are equally important, there is sufficient data available with respect to some components (for example, immunization), and hardly any for other elements (health promotion, parent counselling, and anticipatory guidance).

According to the Working Party, it is possible to check whether the tests, examinations and/or other procedures with respect to secondary prevention, early detection of diseases, disorders and defects by means of (for example) screening, are valid on the basis of existing criteria. The British Working Party has worked this out. In doing so, it defined screening as follows: 'the presumptive identification of unrecognized disease or defect by the application of tests, examinations and other procedures which can be rapidly applied' (Macfarlane et al. 1989). Screening and periodic health examinations form part of what is called a 'Child Health Surveillance Programme'. 'Surveillance involves a set of activities which are initiated by professionals. It includes the oversight of the physical, social, and emotional health and development of all children; measurement and recording of physical growth; monitoring of developmental progress; offering and arranging intervention when necessary; prevention of disease by immunization and other means; and health education (Hall 1989).

The British Joint Working Party has analysed all the screening tests used in the Child Health Care system. The well-known principles of Wilson and

---

[12]The general practitioner can be compared with the Dutch huisarts and the clinical medical officer corresponds to the Dutch CB-arts (doctor who works in a Child Health Clinic). There is no Dutch equivalent for the child health visitor, but this can probably best be compared to a wijkverpleegkundige (district nurse) specialized in Child Health Care.

Jungner (1968), and Cochrane and Holland (1969) were used as a touchstone. The tests and/or procedures that passed this scrutiny were included in the core programme that is set out below. For the early detection of those diseases, defects and disorders for which, according to the Working Party, no valid examination/test exists (as yet), history-taking and clinical observation are used. This applies, for example in the case of developmental disorders and visual disorders (Hall 1989). These examinations and procedures have also been included in the core programme set out below[13].

The main features of this programme are:

Neonatal examination	Review of family history, pregnancy and birth
	Discuss any concerns expressed by parents
	Full physical examination, including weight and head circumference
	Check for congenital dislocation of the hips
	Check for testicular descent
	Inspect eyes
	Examine eyes for red reflex
	If high risk of hearing defect – refer for further testing
6–8 days	Blood tests for phenylketonuria and hypothyroidism
At discharge or within 10 days of birth	Check for congenital dislocation of the hips again
6–8 weeks	Check history and ask about parental concerns
	Physical examination, weight and head circumference
	Check for congenital dislocation of the hips again
	If status of testicular descent not known from birth information, or if not fully descended at birth – check again

---

[13]The Child Health Surveillance Programme in the United Kingdom applies up to the age of 5 years (school entry). The last consultation takes place at this transition. This consultation is not mentioned in the list below: compared with the Dutch situation, it belongs in the Child Health Care programme for 4–19-year-olds.

	Specifically enquire about parental concerns regarding hearing and vision Inspect the eyes Consider giving parents check-list or questionnaire for detection of hearing loss
3 months	Immunization
5 months	Immunization
7–9 months	Enquire about parental concerns regarding health and development Ask specifically about vision and hearing Check weight if indicated or parents wish it Check for congenital dislocation of the hips Check for testicular descent if not previously recorded as being fully down Observe visual behaviour and look for squint Carry out distraction test for hearing Immunization
13 months	Immunization
18–24 months	Enquire about parental concerns, particularly regarding behaviour, vision and hearing Confirm that the child is walking with a normal gait Confirm that the child is beginning to say words and is understanding when spoken to No formal testing of vision and hearing but arrange detailed assessment if there is any doubt about either being normal
36–42 months	Ask about vision, squint, hearing, behaviour and development If any concerns, discuss with the parents whether the child is likely to have special educational needs and arrange further action as appropriate Measure height and plot on centile chart Check for testicular descent unless previously fully descended at birth If there are any concerns about the child's hearing, perform or arrange for a hearing test

Source: Macfarlane, A., Sefi, S., Cordeiro, M.: *Child Health. The screening tests,* Oxford, 1989.

8.4 Similarities and differences between the Netherlands and the United Kingdom

As is shown by the above outlines, the programmes for periodic health examination that were recently recommended in the two countries differ greatly. The main differences concern the content and frequency (what must be checked in each child and when), and the organization of the clinics (open or by appointment). Moreover, the British programme quite explicitly highlights the responsibility and the active role of parents.

8.4.1 Content and frequency

A first major difference between the British and the Dutch situation is that in the United Kingdom, extensive neonatal examination is considered part of Child Health Surveillance, and is recorded as such. It thus provides the basis for further child health care[14]. Of course, all children are examined immediately after birth in the Netherlands too. However, there is no fixed protocol and the expertise of the various examiners differs[15]. Besides, there is a problem in the Netherlands with respect to the transfer of the data of the neonatal examination to the Child Health Care system: the inclusion of these data in the Child Health Care (Jeugdgezondheidszorg JGZ) file is not always streamlined. For British Child Health Surveillance it is recommended that, in addition to the neonatal examination, a limited core programme of tests (screenings) be carried out on children of a certain age. In addition to this screening programme, the child's history is taken at each session and the parents are asked if there is anything about the health or development of the child that they are concerned about. Specific tests are only done on those children in whom this is called for.

The main difference as compared with the recommended programme of the Working Party on PHE (werkgroep PGO) for the Netherlands is that the Dutch programme has a far greater number of predetermined check ups and test items. Following the PKU/CHT screening, parents are asked to

---

[14]Neonatal examination in the United Kingdom comprises the following: 'Weight, head circumference, skin (for colour, birthmarks, etc.), head shape, fontanelles, ears, eye appearance (including red reflex), palate (hard and soft), heart (auscultation), pulses, respiratory system, abdomen, umbilicus, genitalia (including descent of testes in boys), limbs (for normal formation, tone and movement), anus (normal appearance), hips (for congenital dislocation)' (Macfarlane et al. 1989).

[15]Neonatal examination in the Netherlands is carried out by different (para)medics: interns, gynaecologists, paediatricians, general practitioners or midwives.

attend eight times in the United Kingdom and 16 times[16] in the Netherlands (up to the age of 3 years and 9 months to 4 years).

8.4.2 Open clinics and the role of parents

Besides the notification schedule, parents in the United Kingdom have the option of going to a Child Health Clinic whenever they are concerned about the health or development of their child (a system of open clinics). Research has shown that parents regularly make use of this facility, particularly during the first year of the child's life. Hart and others report an average of 10 visits, in addition to the notification schedule (Hart et al. 1981). Allied to the British concept of open clinics is the vision of the British Working Party with respect to the central role of the parents where the health of their children is concerned; it is felt that, in the past, the active role of the parents was not properly acknowledged. According to the British Working Party, 'parents and professionals have to become partners in the care programme, and in all matters that have to do with the health needs of their children'. This is one reason why it is recommended that the child's health record should be in the possession of the parents. The observations of parents are considered to constitute an extremely valuable contribution to the surveillance programme (Macfarlane 1989). So far, attitudes in the Dutch Child Health Care system have been rather sceptical about the role ascribed to parents in the United Kingdom. The lack of insight into the reliability of parent information probably has a lot to do with this. Moreover, the need to reassure parents (in answer to the question: 'Is my child healthy, and if so, is it as healthy as possible?') is highly rated among Dutch Child Health Care professionals. While, in the United Kingdom, parents can consult a doctor when they are concerned about their child, the system in the Netherlands is such that there are frequent contacts with the parents to prevent a situation developing in which parents become worried about the health and/or development of their child.

In summary, the main differences between the (proposed) Dutch programme and the British programme are as follows.

The Netherlands

A frequent notification schedule, care is highly-structured, but (as yet) standardized only to a limited extent. The implementation of neonatal examination and the transfer of the results to the Child Health Care has not

---

[16]When sessions are combined, the total number of times that parents are asked to attend can be reduced to 14; see footnote 8.

yet been formalized. Basically, there are no open clinics exclusively for Child Health Care (although many clinical teams have set up facilities for telephone enquiries).

United Kingdom

Extensive neonatal examination as part of Child Health Surveillance. A far less frequent notification schedule, care is less structured (limited notification schedule in addition to open clinics), but the core programme has been virtually fully standardized.

8.4.3 The possibilities for comparison

The differences mentioned here are interesting because they reflect the discussions that have been going on for a number of years with respect to: the organization of the Dutch periodic health examination concerning the frequency of the notification schedule; the implementation of the neonatal examination; the recording of the results of this examination in the Child Health Care file; the role of parents; and the open clinic. The fact that a new form of organization and content has been realized in a number of districts in the United Kingdom, now makes empirical comparison of the two systems possible. Of course, the first question to ask is: to what extent are the two systems comparable, considering the different organizational and epidemiological contexts of the Dutch and British health care systems? A second question is whether the differences are as great in practice as the ideal programmes would suggest. One might, for example, assume that the total number of visits that parents pay to consultatiebureaus or Child Health Clinics does not differ very much: parents who are seldom called up may well make frequent use of open clinics. In view of the fact that there is practically no data on outcomes available for either of the systems, it would seem evident that a study should be done on this aspect[17]. Such a study should answer the following questions:

- Taking into account the different organizational and epidemiological contexts of the Dutch and British systems of Child Health Care, is it possible to compare the two programmes in terms of quality, effects, and costs?

---

[17]As mentioned above in footnote 2, the recommendations of Hall (1989) have by no means been realized in all Health Districts (see Donkers & Merkx 1990). Of course, the same applies for the recommendations of the Dutch Working Party on periodic health examinations.

- If so, can any indications be given in the light of possible differences in quality, effects and costs, of the advantages and disadvantages of the two systems, for example, with respect to the desirable extent of structuring and standardization?

- With respect to the desirable extent of structuring, the question of whether the open clinics in the United Kingdom meet, prevent or actually generate a need for care must also be answered. To this end, the study should chart the total consumption of care for children, including the care provided outside the Child Health Care system, in both the United Kingdom and the Netherlands.

- In measuring the effect of parental responsibility, which serves as an important point of departure for the programme in the United Kingdom, the target groups that attend the open clinics should also be looked at: if only the 'worried well' come to the clinics, and not the persons at risk, then the real target group is not being reached.

Within the framework of the Project on the Integral Evaluation of Child Health Care (Project Integrale Evaluatie Jeugdgezondheidszorg), NIPG/ TNO has been requested to formulate a proposal for a study to answer these questions.

Finally, the Utrecht Research Centre for Child Health Care and Child Welfare (Centrum voor Onderzoek en Ontwikkeling van Jeugdgezond-heidszorg) at the University of Utrecht is preparing a study on the role of parents. This study will focus on the question what Dutch parents (for example, in comparison with their British counterparts) think of the way in which their responsibility for the health of their children is reflected within the pre-school Child Health Care system, The advantages and disadvan-tages of the so-called parent-held record will also be discussed[18].

8.5 Recommendations

- The Project Group recommends that the term periodic medical examination in pre-school Child Health Care be replaced by periodic health examination in accordance with the definition given in this chapter.

---

[18]In addition to the parent-held record, British doctors also keep their own records; this means that there is a double system of administration (Seminar: Health for All Children, London, 17 January 1992; Verloove 1992, personal communication).

- The Project Group recommends that, within the framework of the further development of a protocol of the periodic health examination, studies on the programme proposed by the Working Party on PHE (Burgmeijer et al. 1991), aimed at feasibility, effectiveness and cost effectiveness, be carried out in one or more trial regions.

- In order to be able to make well-considered decisions regarding the desired frequency, the degree of structuring and standardization of the periodic health examination, it is desirable that, in addition to the study mentioned in the second recommendation, a comparative study be done on the Dutch and British periodic health examination programmes, as indicated in section 8.4.3.

References

Burgmeijer, R.J.F., Boeken Kruger-Mangunkusumo, R.S., Fernandes, J. (red.): *Periodiek geneeskundig onderzoek. Een praktijkboek voor de jeugd-gezondheidszorg*, Utrecht: Bunge, 1991.

Butler, J.: *Child Health Surveillance in Primary Care. A critical Review*, London: Department of Health, 1989.

Chatab, J.: *Consultatiebureau-teams in beeld*, Utrecht: NIVEL, 1989.

Cochrane, A. & Holland, W.: Validation of screening procedures, *British Medical Bulletin* 27 (1969) 3–8.

Cuisinier, M.C.J. & Jonkers, R.: Onderzoek en protocolontwikkeling bij patiëntenvoorlichting, *Tijdschrift Sociale Gezondheidszorg* 64 (1986) 2, 34–37.

Donkers, L. & Merkx, J.: *How to arrange less?*, Leiden: NIPG/TNO, 1990.

Gezondheidsraad: *Jaaradvies gezondheidszorg 1990*, Den Haag 1990.

Hall, D.M.B. (ed.): *Health for all children. A Programme for Child Health Surveillance*, Oxford: Oxford University Press, 1989.

Hart, H., Bax, M., Jenkins, S.: Use of the child health clinic, *Archives of Disease in Childhood* 56 (1981) 440–445.

Jonge, G.A. de: Redactioneel, *Tijdschrift voor Jeugdgezondheidszorg* 24 (1992) 1, 2.

Macfarlane, J.A. & Pillay, U.: Who does what and how much in the preschool child health services in England, *British Medical Journal* 289 (1984), 851–852 .

Macfarlane, A., Sefi, S., Cordeiro, M.: *Child Health. The screening tests*, Practical Guides for General Practice 11, Oxford: Oxford Medical Publications, 1989.

Mcfarlane, J.A.: Lessen uit de Engelse jeugdgezondheidszorg, in: Bos, M.W. & Winter, M. de (red.): *Jeugdgezondheidszorg in de toekomst*, Lisse: Swets & Zeitlinger, 1989, pp.113–119.

Nederlandse Vereniging voor Jeugdgezondheidszorg: *De Jeugdgezondheidszorg in 2000; Beleidsplan*, Utrecht 1990.

Vissers, T.C.G.M.: Protocollaire Geneeskunde, *Medisch Contact* 23 (1983) 685–688.

Wilson, J.M.G. & Jungner, G.: *Principles and practice of screening for disease*, (Public Health Papers 34), Geneve: WHO, 1968.

Further reading

Nationale Raad voor de Volksgezondheid: *Advies inzake de versterking van de preventie in de eerstelijnszorg*, Zoetermeer: NRV-publ. 6/92, 1992.

9 Prevention of psychosocial and educational problems

The promotion of optimal psychosocial development and the promotion of good parent-child relationships constitute a major part of pre-school Child Health Care work. Distinguishing signs that point to disorders and/or problems in this field is one of the objectives of this type of care. In the social context such attention is certainly called for: parents have a lot of questions on development and upbringing and want support and professional advice from the clinical team (Kousemaker et al. 1987). Various recommendations made by or to the Government (National Committee for Early Detection 1988, Youth Policy Council; see: Raad voor het Jeugdbeleid 1986, Ministry of Welfare, Public Health and Cultural Affairs 1992) argue for increased efforts in these fields by pre-school Child Health Care. These recommendations usually consider pre-school Child Health Care to be an important 'finding place' for psychosocial developmental disorders and educational problems, and to be one of the readily accessible facilities in which problems can be spotted at an early stage and counselling or referral given where needed. Parental trust in pre-school Child Health Care and high coverage are held to be major advantages. Within pre-school Child Health Care, there are various working methods to tackle such problems. At visits to the clinic, psychosocial development and upbringing are recurring themes. These matters are often discussed during examinations, for instance that with the Van Wiechen check-list[1] or the periodic health examination. Sometimes parents ask explicit questions, or they indicate implicitly that they are worried or have problems. Nurses and Clinical Medical Officers, sometimes supported by educational counsellors, give 'anticipatory guidance' during home visits, clinics and/or group meetings: information on possible problems that in specific stages of development may present themselves, either with the child or in the parent-child relationship. If problems that cannot be solved by some simple advice are identified by the parents or by the clinical team, there are several options for short-term guidance. More severe problems are always referred.

---

[1]Partly based on the Denver Developmental Scale, the Van Wiechen check-list was developed in the early 1980s to promote the systematic examination of development (motor development, language and speech, personality and social behaviour) and to achieve uniform national registration. For details see Chapter 6, section 5.

Some elements of the working methods described above can be characterized as standardized programmed prevention. This applies notably to the developmental examination making use of the Van Wiechen check-list, in which psychosocial development plays a major part (see Chapter 6). The Early Detection language test discussed in Chapter 7 may be considered important in identifying aspects of psychosocial problems[2]. These problems will not be discussed explicitly in this chapter. The majority of the procedures mentioned here can be classified as prevention to measure, or even as non-specific oversight (Butler 1989). They are forms of prevention and care arising from the regular contacts between parents and the team of the clinic, the major instruments being the knowledge, experience and preventive clinical eye of the medical officers and nurses. Of course, this individually focused working method poses a problem for outcome assessment. As already indicated in this report it is exactly this very important form of prevention that is hardest to express in measures and numbers. In this chapter, references in scientific literature to the nature and prevalence of psychosocial and educational problems are first reviewed. Subsequently, existing and experimental working methods relating to these problems are highlighted; then it is considered what possibilities and problems present themselves in examining the effectiveness of psychosocial and teaching prevention activities. Attention is also paid to a prevention model. The chapter is concluded with conclusions and recommendations.

9.1 Psychosocial problems

There is some ambiguity about the definition and classification of psychosocial problems with children. Verhulst (1985) argues that the ambiguities are inherent to the subject: it is about the behaviour of children. A child's behaviour cannot be detached from its development phase. There should be consensus on the types of behaviour that can be considered normal for a given age group. In addition to this, a child's behaviour is situational (it results from the transactions between the child and its environment), but also personal (there is great diversity in behaviour of children of the same age). The assessment of childlike behaviour also has a strongly subjective component: it is grown-ups (parents or experts) who assess specific behaviour as problematic or deviant. The adult's individual standards will always play a part, but so will social and cultural standards. These standards may, however, vary on the grounds of individual

---

[2]Communicative development is a major aspect of psychosocial development and may act as an indicator of disorders/problems in other domains of psychosocial development.

characteristics and socio-cultural aspects. When parents call certain behaviour by their child problematic or deviant, this has to do with their own views on how children should behave at a certain age, and with their own and their family's resilience.

On the other hand, the experts may also call certain behaviour problematic on the basis of more objective professional knowledge and/or experience with many children. On this basis, an expert can assess whether specific behaviour is common, or exceptional (and therefore deviant or problematic). Among scientists, but also in society as a whole however, there are different notions about what is to be considered normal behaviour and what is considered pathological and/or problematic behaviour. Problematic/pathological behaviour may be caused by a neurophysiological disorder but also by relational problems or incompetence of parents or guardians. Usually, however, several factors play a part in the development and the course of such disorders and/or problems.

The lack of clarity described above makes itself felt at the level of research into these problems among (small) children. American and British epidemiological investigations give values for prevalence ranging from 6% to 50% (Koot & Verhulst 1991). Vagueness in definitions and classification hamper comparison of the results of these investigations. On the basis of the CBCL/2–3 (Child Behaviour Checklist for ages 2–3) Koot & Verhulst (1991) recently did epidemiological research into the incidence of behavioural and emotional problems among 2-year-olds and 3-year-olds in the Netherlands. The investigation shows that much of the behaviour experienced as problematic by parents is found in over half the population of children this age. Such behaviour is usually developmental and should not be interpreted as pathological. It is rare that isolated problematic behaviour indicates psychopathology. Combinations of types of problematic behaviour, however, may well be an indication for psychopathology. Koot and Verhulst report that 7.8% of the children examined show problematic behaviour that may be called pathological.

9.2 Educational problems

There is ambiguity too about the definition and classification of child-rearing problems. Though questions and problems of child-rearing are of all times, it is clear that they have received ever more (professional) attention in the last few years. This increase in attention and supply should be based on an increased demand from the parents. From various investigations it emerges that parents are feeling more and more uncertain about child-rearing (Youth Policy Council; see: Raad voor het Jeugdbeleid

1986, Kousemaker et al. 1987, Wilbrink-Griffioen & Van Eijck 1990). These investigations advance many causes for an increase in problems (and therefore in uncertainty). The decrease in family size has resulted in an increasing number of parents having little personal experience of the growth and development of children. Moreover, the child has to attain adulthood in an ever more complex and ever faster changing society; what is traditionally passed on by parents to adolescents is often no longer applicable or no longer satisfactory. The family has become more isolated and family ties have loosened; the possibility of a conscious choice for parenthood is often accompanied by great expectations with regard to parenthood, which increase the chance of disappointment and generate more tension and uncertainty. An accumulation of such factors may result in educational problems which parents are incapable of handling.

A fairly recent attempt at classification was made by Kousemaker and Timmers-Huigens (1985). They designed a classification of educational situations according to the severity of the problem: ordinary educational situation; educational tension; educational crisis; and problematic child-rearing situation. The characteristics of the different stages are based on experience in primary and secondary care. According to Wilbrink-Griffioen & Van Eijck (1990), further empirical foundation is as yet lacking. This classification may serve a useful purpose in the division of tasks between different (care) agencies which are concerned with these problems.

At present, there is little clarity regarding the influence and character of the factors which play a part in the process of bringing up children. The transactional model of thought that has been used in the last few years (see also Chapter 6), makes it possible to examine the influence of the various factors. This model is based on three categories of factors working in continuous interaction:

- child factors (personality traits, disposition, aptitude, intelligence, physical condition, looks, age, stage of development and competence)

- parental factors (personality, biography, educational targets, intelligence, perception of and competence in parenthood, attitude towards the child, expectations, style of upbringing)

- environmental factors (working conditions, housing, presence of a social support network, occurrence of stressful life-events[3]).

However, the breadth of the model at the same time constitutes its

---

[3]Generally stressful life-events are taken to mean: death of relatives of friends, divorce, moving house, change in employment and so on.

weakness: the number of possible combinations is so large that predictions on the development or the course of a problem of upbringing are hard to make. An advantage of the transactional model of thought is that attention is not only paid to risk factors (such as the above mentioned stressful life-events), but also to protective factors (*inter alia* Garmezy & Rutter 1983, Groenendaal et al. 1987). Major protective factors mentioned are: competence or fighting spirit (the feeling of being capable of handling a situation and solving problems), coping (capacity for handling and coming to terms with tension) and a social support system (a supportive network of relatives, friends, acquaintances, neighbours and colleagues) (*inter alia* Bosma & Hosman 1990). The above approach provides starting-points for prevention: 'Attention is indicated for the child as well as for the parent, for the environment and for protective factors such as increasing the fighting spirit and the presence of support from a network of relatives and friends. Finally attention should be paid to the influence of tensions related to the children's ages and the so-called stressful life-events' (Wilbrink-Griffioen & Van Eijck 1990).

Until now, little research has been done in the Netherlands into the prevalence of educational problems. When considering prevalence, a distinction should be made between on the one hand problems for which professional help is called in (or would be required) and on the other hand questions or problems (tensions) which really arise in every upbringing, but about which parents nevertheless ask for advice and guidance. From the investigation by Kousemaker et al. (1987), 74% of mothers with children in the birth–4 years age group (and notably the 1.5–4 years group) proved to have questions concerning the upbringing of their children; problems most often mentioned are obstinacy and disobedience. Other figures are used to estimate the prevalence of educational problems: Wilbrink-Griffioen and Van Eijck (1990) make use of Regional Institutes for Ambulant Mental Health Care (RIAGG) registration figures (in 1986, 5000 children between birth and 6 years) and the research results from Verhulst (1985) on severe psychic disorders among 8–11-year-olds (7%) and moderate to severe disorders in the same age group (19%). The Ministry of Welfare, Public Health and Cultural Affairs in its memorandum *Educational Support to Measure* (Opvoedingssteun op maat) also gives figures on minor or severe problems among young people (10–25%[4]). On the prevalence of these problems the memorandum states: Some 5–10% of parents of young children say they experience considerable problems with upbringing. Without commitment, because of the lack of a general overview, the prevalence of severe emotional and behavioural problems with young people in the Netherlands may be estimated at 5–7%' (SCP 1987) (Ministry of Welfare, Public Health and Cultural Affairs 1992). From these data, it

---

[4]Verhulst (1985), Deboutte (1989) and Van der Linden & Dijkman (1989).

appears that in the research done so far, the extent of (psychosocial) problems with children and the extent to which parents report having difficulties with their children's upbringing cannot easily be distinguished between.

9.3 Working methods in pre-school Child Health Care

Right from the time the well-baby clinics were founded, parental questions and problems with respect to child-rearing have been given attention. This is done both during regular sessions of the clinics and during home visits by the district nurse. The local Community Health Care services have, in addition, deployed many initiatives, such as group clinics, group education, counselling by educationalists in a clinic and the development of toddler information leaflets[5]. The regular package of pre-school Child Health Care in this field includes home visits by district nurses, information for (prospective) parents and anticipatory guidance on the basis of physical examination and parental questions. The field of the prevention of psychosocial and educational problems is certainly not the exclusive terrain of the Community Health Care however; many other agencies are also experimenting in this field. In many cases there is cooperation between a number of organizations, including the Community Health Care, the Municipal Health Services Departments for Child Health Care for 4–19-year-olds, Childline, Health and Education, the Ambulant Mental Health Care (RIAGGs) and community youth welfare networks. An overview of the 97 projects set up in this field is given in the report on the investigation *Preventie van opvoedingsproblemen by 0–12 jarigen* (Prevention of Educational Problems between birth and the age of 12) (Wilbrink-Griffioen & Van Eijck 1990). It is characteristic of many of these projects that they can be placed between primary and secondary care. They are particularly aimed at parents and children who have to contend with problems marginally too serious for primary care (Community Health Care for example) but yet not serious enough for secondary care (such as provided by RIAGGs).

As stated in the introduction to this chapter, the majority of the activities in this field can be classified as prevention to measure. The objective, however, of many of the projects mentioned above is to give a number of these activities (notably anticipatory information and the identifying of problems and disorders) a more standardized character by means of thorough research into the causes of disorders and problems and thorough research

---

[5]Toddler information leaflets are folders with age-specific information on the development of the child. Subjects include: eating, sleeping, play, behaviour, toilet training, obstinacy.

on outcome measures. Short-term assistance for minor problems and referral for more severe problems are by nature forms of prevention to measure.

9.4 Scientific state-of-the-art

9.4.1 Outcome measures

The objective of prevention of psychosocial and educational problems was said in the introduction to be on the one hand the prevention of such problems and on the other hand the early identification of psychosocial disorders and educational problems. The objective is attained through: anticipatory guidance; and early identification of problems. Early identification of problems can be followed up by either short-term assistance (for minor problems) or referral (for more serious problems).

For the purpose of evaluating the above activities the following outcome measures may be formulated.

- Anticipatory guidance about age group problems: the health professional at the clinic anticipates problems that he/she knows arise more often in specific age groups, for instance eating problems, obstinacy and the like. He/she will give advice/information on how to act when these problems occur. The effect of this counselling can be measured against greater parental skill (knowledge) and competence (action) with regard to age-specific problems and against the improvement of the parent-child relationship.

- (Early) identification of problems: the professional at the clinic and/or the parents identify problems: there are two possibilities:
  (a) Short-term guidance from the clinic (either by clinical medical officer or district nurse or by a teacher) in case of minor problems. The effect of the identification can be measured against parental competence in learning to cope with the problematic behaviour and against the satisfaction of the parents concerned with the advice received. Parental satisfaction indicates that they can apply the advice received (it is practicable), and that in the opinion of those concerned it is effective.
  (b) Referral in case of more serious problems; these are problems of such a nature that more comprehensive counselling and/or treatment seems necessary.
  The effect of the identification can in this case be measured against the success of the referral: that is to say that parents and child

reach the right (secondary care) channel and that there the referral is found to be justified.

The outcome measures referred to are called intermediate outcome measures which enable a first pronouncement to be made (in the short term) on the effectiveness of the methods employed. There are differing views on the necessity, desirability and feasibility of short-term versus long-term outcome measures.

Bosma & Hosman (1990), in their study into the susceptibility of the determinants of psychical health to influence, recommend not restricting the evaluation to intermediate (short term) outcome measures. The use of intermediate outcome measures (such as the raising of parental competence), so they say, is justified only if increased parental competence is proven to have a positive effect on the psychosocial development and mental health of the children. Their analysis further shows that positive effects are more likely to be found in the long term than in the short term. Wilbrink-Griffioen (1989) on the other hand holds that it is not practicable to legitimize prevention of educational problems purely on the basis of the long-term effect and the prevention of serious problems. 'The yield had better be measured against short-term objectives and related to the range of the intervention' (Wilbrink-Griffioen 1989). She mentions possible objectives including: increasing parental child-rearing skills; enlarging informal networks; and decreasing the number of referrals to special schools. In addition to this, it can be justifiably asked whether it is possible, from the point of view of the transactional development model, to prove unequivocally the effectiveness of a educationally preventive activity in the short term as well as in the long term. Making the effectiveness operational might cause problems as well: will the effect be a decreasing use of youth welfare services? It might just as well be an increase in demand.

In the Netherlands, it may be finally observed, there has been hardly any research into the effectiveness of the prevention of educational problems.

9.4.2 Problems in outcome measurement

One of the problems in evaluating activities in the field of psychosocial and educational problem prevention is the ambiguity in definition and classification mentioned above. The notion of psychosocial and educational problems is hard to define with precision. This broad term covers problems that lie closer to the medical/psychiatric term disorder as well as problems lying closer to the social notion of conflict. This makes the notion psychosocial and educational problems ambiguous: it relates to departures from both the medical norm and the social norm (Van Gennep 1991).

An additional problem is that this field is the object of three separate and mutually independent disciplines: child psychiatry and developmental psychology deal with (problematic) child behaviour, and educationalists with educational problems (which may have been caused by problematic child behaviour). Each discipline has its point of view and its own theoretical concept or concepts. According to current scientific opinion (the transactional development model, see Chapter 6) a child's social development is inextricably bound up with the way the parents bring it up. Knowledge and understanding of problems that may arise and the possibilities for preventive interventions demand close cooperation of the disciplines mentioned. As can be deduced from the above it is not, or practically not, possible to separate the problematic behaviour of children on the one hand and the educational problems of the parents on the other. These problems are usually interchangeable; for instance no clear distinction is made in research into prevalence.

Hardly any research data are available with reference to the outcome of anticipatory guidance. The few investigations into outcome carried out abroad (Gutelius et al. 1977, Chamberlain et al. 1979, 1980, Dworkin et al. 1987) show divergent results. Little research has been carried out so far in the Netherlands either. The toddler information leaflets project (Boost et al. 1991) is an exception. The objective of the leaflets is to contribute to maintaining or achieving a satisfactory educational situation. A poll among parents (response 30%, some 300 parents) gave the following results: 96% read the leaflets mainly for the feeling of recognition and the useful tips. A large number of parents (70%) were also reassured by the text. The leaflets further stimulated a large number of parents (70%) to discuss education with others (partner, friends, relatives); it induced some 10% to start a discussion on upbringing with the clinical team.

A little more research has been done on the early recognition of psychosocial problems with children, although there are very divergent ideas on the possibilities. Opponents stress that current scientific understanding of the problem (knowledge of aetiology, natural course, prevalence and incidence and so on) is not sufficient to develop Early Detection methods. Thus Gerards (1985) interprets the available research data as not scientifically warranting an unqualified choice for Early Detection of psychosocial disorders or problems. Many psychosocial disorders are believed to recover spontaneously and psychosocial disorders in children are considered to be of little or no prognostic value with reference to future mental health. Early Detection is acceptable for psychosocial disorders with a large chance of continuity. This however presupposes more specific and reliable knowledge of the natural course of various types of disorders, knowledge that is not yet available. Advocates of Early Detection in this field, Hosman (1987) for one, argue that, notwithstanding limited understanding of psychosocial disorders, enough is known about the causes of such problems to justify Early Detection activities. Within the group of Early Detection proponents there are experts who think the best way of detecting psychosocial disorders is by means of anamnesis and observation; others argue in favour of a more standardized method, for instance a behavioural questionnaire, because they hold the view that clinical judgement is subjective by definition (Dohrenwend et al. 1971, Elstein 1976, Earls et al. 1982).

In the past, various questionnaires were developed with the intention of effecting a first division in a general population of children between those with and without disturbed behaviour (Willoughby & Haggerty 1964, Richman et al. 1982, Verhulst & Akkerhuis 1983). Earls et al. (1982) investigated the suitability for screening purposes of the Behavioural Screenings Questionnaire (BSQ) developed by Richman et al. (1982) for the purpose of an epidemiological study into behavioural problems with 3-year-olds. The investigators say in conclusion: '...this parent report method appears to function satisfactorily as a screening instrument, although the limits of its generalizability in different cultural contexts must be regarded cautiously' (Earls et al. 1982). Verhulst and Akkerhuis (1983), who translated the latter part of the BSQ (the part specifically dealing with behaviour) reach a similar conclusion after research. This opinion is not shared by the British Joint Working Party on Child Health Surveillance (Hall 1989). With reference to outcome assessment of screening within Child Health Surveillance in Britain they argue that insufficient scientific research has been done to introduce the BSQ for routine screening. They think such questionnaires may be useful as check-lists in discussions on behavioural problems between the clinical medical officer or district nurse and parents, or as an aid for parents in recognizing behavioural problems in their children.

9.5 First step towards a prevention model

Wilbrink-Griffioen and Van Eijck (1990), in their extensive investigation into the prevention of problems of upbringing, attempted to draw up a model for successful prevention activities. They did so on the basis of national and international research data. With reference to the projects abroad they concluded that a number of elements contribute to the success of such projects:

• parental involvement

- close cooperation of parents and professionals

- transfer of responsibility to the parents, which proves to be a way of enhancing interest, motivation and participation

- home visits, which make those concerned feel that there is real interest in their problems

- the possibility to continue the newly learned activities at home; parents prefer to see immediate results from what they have learned; therefore it makes sense to learn activities that can be applied at once;

- an approach involving a larger community, for instance one focused on a district with cooperation between the various agencies

- several agencies working on the same project widens its range

- attention paid to the prenatal and perinatal periods.

Concerning national projects, they observe in the first place that, even though a variety of activities is being developed by the existing network of facilities (see section 9.3), there is little coherence and method at local and neighbourhood levels. 'The work done is hardly ever based on epidemiological data. This was apparent to us in *inter alia* the numerous reports and studies concerning the methods applied. Usually these are undergraduates' dissertations which are hardly comparable with one another. Neither has it proved possible to formulate a research plan which will make the outcome of a preventive activity operational. Method in reporting and concrete testing of the objective is usually lacking...On the basis of existing reporting it can hardly be ascertained, what methods are in effect most suitable for the prevention of educational problems' (Wilbrink-Griffioen and Van Eijck 1990). The broad conclusions to be drawn in regard to the conditions for a successful course of projects include:

- Projects aimed at parents and children should as far as possible be targeted on one neighbourhood and set up in a familiar and accessible location (such as the clinic)

- A community focus promotes the cooperation between various agencies working on education in a district (networking)

- Information on the raising and development of children should be tangible, practical and focused on one subject.

On the basis of all these data, a model was constructed for the prevention of educational problems. A central role was given to a youth welfare community network; this network lies between, on the one hand, zero care and primary care facilities which attend to support, information, identification and minor help and care, and on the other hand, the secondary care organizations and cooperating agencies that can be called upon, if required, to provide diagnostics and assistance. 'These networks offer the possibilities of:

- using all agencies concerned with the birth–12-year-olds
- developing individual and collective prevention strategies
- paying attention, geared to the specific problems of a community, to special risk groups
- fulfilling all the teaching preventive functions described and linking up with the Early Detection organizations and the facilities for youth welfare' (Wilbrink-Griffioen & Van Eijck 1990).

In this connection, it should be said that, the effect of a strategy targeted on risk groups is also doubted (De Boer & Schmitz 1987).

9.6 Conclusions

In this specific phase of child development (the pre-school period) attention paid to educational and psychosocial problems is of great importance. The need for support in this field is apparent, among other things from the numerous questions confronting district nurses and clinical medical officers. Pre-school Child Health Care in particular can play a large part in the early identification of and counselling on psychosocial and educational problems.

Although in the practice of pre-school Child Health Care there is no lack of interest in this field, there is not yet a good conceptual framework from which these activities can be initiated and evaluated. Activities in the field could be made systematic, and effective identification and counselling methods should be developed for children's psychosocial problems and for parental uncertainty on questions of upbringing. In short, many activities up till now tailored to individual situations lend themselves to a more standardized approach. It should be noted however, that an individually tailored approach is usually the most appropriate: it is precisely the familiar contact between parents and professionals as established in pre-school Child Health Care that is a condition for the identification of problems parents do not talk about readily or easily. A standardized approach certainly does not exclude prevention to measure. On the contrary, the two forms should be seen as complementary.

The possibilities of a more standardized approach are being investigated by *inter alia* the Pedagogic Department of Utrecht State University. Their research concerns the development of identification and counselling methods for psychosocial and educational problems, aiming at further systematizing both the support of parents in their task of child-rearing and the early identification of minor to serious psychosocial problems (Groenendaal & Rispens 1991). The method to be developed is based on a model of family pressures (after Robbroeckx & Wels 1988).

Supporting parents in the upbringing and the psychosocial development of their children is an integral part of pre-school Child Health Care work. Anticipatory information and early identification of problems are the major tools in this context and are closely interwoven with practically all the components of care. Parents appeared to appreciate the support and supply of information, as is evident from the many questions asked about psychosocial and educational problems in pre-school Child Health Care. There is also a great demand for this aspect from society as a whole, as is evident from the important part ascribed to Child Health Care in the context of educational support and prevention of psychosocial problems (Ministry of Welfare, Public Health and Cultural Affairs 1992). Research, however, shows that much remains to be done in the field of promoting expertise. Further systematizing of methods in this field, as indicated above, may well be of great help.

9.7 Recommendations

- The Project Group take the view that early identification of educational and psychosocial problems and support for parents (by means of anticipatory information, for instance) constitutes an integral element of pre-school Child Health Care. Quality improvement in this field should especially be effected by means of promoting expertise, clear task descriptions and further systematizing of methods.

- The Project Group attach great value to close cooperation and coordination with other agencies that target on prevention and aid in the field of psychosocial and educational problems. As appears from sections 9.3 and 9.5 there are a large number of agencies active in this field. In the policy memorandum of the Ministry of Welfare, Public Health and Cultural Affairs (1992) *Opvoedingssteun op maat* (Educational Support to Measure) the cooperation between various agencies is specifically given high priority.

References

Boer, F. de & Schmitz, L.: *Risico-groepen en Preventie in de Ambulante Geestelijke Gezondheidszorg*, Utrecht 1987.

Boost, E., Lim-Feyen, J.F., Velzen-Mol, H.W.M. van, Copier, C., Koornneef, N., Akkermans, J.: De Peuterbrief; hulpmiddel in de pedagogische preventie, *Tijdschrift voor Jeugdgezondheidszorg* 23 (1991) 6, 87–89.

Bosma, M.W.M., Hosman, C.M.H.: *Preventie op waarde geschat. Een studie naar de beïnvloedbaarheid van determinanten van psychische gezondheid*, Meppel 1990.

Butler, J.R.: *Child Health Surveillance in Primary Care; A critical review*, London 1989.

Chamberlain, R.W., Szumowski, E.K., Zastowmy, T.R.: An evaluation of efforts to educate mothers about child development and pediatric office practices, *American Journal of Public Health* 69 (1979) 875–886.

Chamberlain, R.W., Szumowski, E.K.: A follow-up study of parent education in pediatric office practices: Impact at age two and a half, *American Journal of Public Health* 70 (1980) 1180 e.v.

Deboutte, D.: *Jeugd en hulp: een psychiatrisch epidemiologische verkenning*, Leuven 1989.

Dohrenwend, B., Egri, B., Mendelsohn, F.: Psychiatric Disorder in general populations: a study of the problem of clinical judgement, *American Journal of Psychiatry* 127 (1971) 1304–1312.

Dworkin, P.H., Allen, D., Geertsma, M.A., Solkoske, L., Cullina, J.: Does developmental content influence the effectiveness of anticipatory guidance?, *Pediatrics* 80 (1987) 196–202.

Earls, F., Jacobs, G., Goldfein, D.S., Silbert, A., Beardslee, W. & Rivinus, T.: Concurrent validation of a behaviour problem scale to use with 3-year-old children, *Journal of the American Academy of Child Psychiatry* 21 (1982) 47–57.

Elstein, A.: Clinical Judgement: Psychological Research and medical practice, *Science* 194 (1976) 696–700.

Garmezy, N. & Rutter, M. (eds.): *Stress, coping, and development in children*, New York 1983.

Gennep, A. van: Preventie van Psychosociale en Pedagogische Problematiek (inleiding), in: *Effectmaten voor de preventieve jeugdgezondheidszorg*, interne publikatie Project Integrale Evaluatie Jeugdgezondheidszorg, Utrecht: Rijksuniversiteit Utrecht, 1991.

Gerards, F.M.: Van kwaad tot erger? De geldigheid van de continuïteits-hypothese in de psychosociale preventie, *Maandblad voor de Geestelijke Volksgezondheid* 3 (1985) 243–258.

Groenendaal, H. et al. (red.): *Protectieve factoren in de ontwikkeling van kinderen en adolescenten*, Lisse 1987.

Groenendaal, J. en Rispens, J.: *Ontwikkeling en evaluatie van een signalerings-en begeleidingsmethodiek van psychosociale problemen en opvoedingsvragen t.b.v. de JGZ 0–4 jaar*, interne publikatie Project Integrale Evaluatie Jeugdgezondheidszorg, Utrecht: Rijksuniversiteit Utrecht, 1991.

Gutelius, M.F., Kirsch, A.D., MacDonald S., et al.: Controlled study of child health supervision. Behavioural results, *Pediatrics* 60 (1977) 294–304.

Hall, D.M.B. (ed.): *Health for All Children; A Programme for Child Health Surveillance*, Oxford 1989.

Hosman, C.M.H.: Effectiviteit van preventieve interventies: mogelijkheden en voorwaarden, in: Schrameijer, F. (red.): *De Nota 2000 ter discussie*, Alphen aan de Rijn 1987, pp. 159–169.

Koot, H.M., Verhulst, F.C.: Prevalence of problem behaviour in Dutch children aged 2–3, *Acta Psychiatrica Scandinavica* 83 (1991) suppl. 367.

Kousemaker, N.P.J & Timmers-Huigens, D.: Pedagogische hulpverlening in de eerste lijn. 'Primaire ambulante jeugdhulpverlening' in pedagogisch perspectief, *Tijdschrift voor Orthopedagogiek* 24 (1985) 549–565.

Kousemaker, N.P.J. et al.: *Pedagogische Preventie in de Jeugdgezondheidszorg voor 0 tot 4 jarigen*, Leiden 1987.

Linden, F.J. van der & Dijkman, T.A.: *Jong zijn en volwassen worden in Nederland*, Nijmegen 1989.

Ministerie van WVC: *Opvoedingssteun op maat. Hoofdlijnen pedagogische preventie in het kader van het jeugdbeleid*, Den Haag 1992.

Nationale Kruisvereniging, *Preventie van Psychosociale en Pedagogische Problematiek door het Kruiswerk; een ontwerpnota*, Bunnik 1988.

Richman, N., Stevenson, J., Graham, P.J.: *Pre-school to school; A Behavioural Study*, London/New York 1982.

Robbroeckx, L.M.H., Wels, P.M.A.: De Nijmeegse vragenlijst voor de opvoedingssituaties, in: Schoorl, P.M., Vries, A.K. de, Wijnekus, M.C. (red.): *Gezinsonderzoek. Methoden in de gezinsdiagnostiek*, Nijmegen 1988.

SCP (Sociaal Cultureel Planbureau): *Samenhang in de zorg voor jeugdigen* (Stukwerk 43), Rijswijk 1987.

Verhulst, F.C., Akkerhuis, G.W.: Gedragsvragenlijst voor driejarigen, *Tijdschrift voor Jeugdgezondheidszorg* 15 (1983) 18–20.

Verhulst, F.C.: *Mental Health in Dutch Children*, Rotterdam 1985 (dissertation).

Wilbrink-Griffioen, D.: Beleid, praktijk en onderzoek. Preventie van opvoedingsproblemen, *Tijdschrift Jeugdonderzoek* sept. (1989) 3, 2–12.

Wilbrink-Griffioen, D. & Eijck, A.M. van: *Preventie van opvoedingsproblemen bij 0–12 jarigen*, Leiden 1990.

Willoughby, J., Haggerty, R.: A simple behaviour questionnaire for preschool children, *Pediatrics* 34 (1964) 798–806.

Further reading

Balledux, M., Mare, J. de, Winter, M. de: *Project Integrale Evaluatie Jeugd-gezondheidszorg voor kinderen van 0–4 jaar. Literatuurstudies*, Utrecht: Rijksuniversiteit Utrecht, 1990.

Gerards, F.M.: *Psychosociale educatie: een strategie voor preventie?; een kritische en theoretische studie over de preventie in de Ambulante Geestelijke Gezondheidszorg*, z.p. 1984 (dissertation).

Liederken, P.C.: De effectiviteit van preventie van psychosociale stoornissen, in: Jonkers, R. et al. (red.): *Effectiviteit van Gezondheidsvoorlichting en opvoeding*, Utrecht 1988, pp. 246–253.

Knops, J.: Preventie van kindermishandeling: tussen droom en werkelijk-heid....., *Het Kind* 4 (1988) 21–23.

Landelijke Commissie VTO: *Een beweging in ontwikkeling; slotadvies*, Rijswijk 1988.

Price, R.H.: *What do successful Prevention Programs have in common?*, Testimony given to the House select Committee, Children, Youth and Families, House of Representatives, U.S. Congress 1987.

Raad voor het Jeugdbeleid: *Opvoeding ondersteund*, Rijswijk 1986.

Robins, L.N.: Antisocial behaviour disturbances of childhood, in: Anthony, E.J. & Koupernik, C. (eds.): *The Child and His Family: Children at Psychiatric Risk*, New York 1974.

Rutter, M., Tizard, J., Whitmore, K.: *Education, health and behaviour*, London 1970.

Ryan, J.M.: Child Abuse and Community Health Nurse, *Home Health Care* 7 (1989) 2, 23–26.

Swaak, A.J., Kousemaker, N.P.J., Wilbrink-Griffioen, D.W.: Consultatiebur-eaus en opvoeding. Een kort selectief verslag van onderzoek in Noord-Brabant,

Tijdschrift voor Jeugdgezondheidszorg 19 (1987) 3, 35–37.

Velden, J. van der: Thema: pedagogische preventie, inleiding, *VTO-nieuwsbrief* 8 (1991) 3/4, 4–5.

Verhulst, F.C., Akkerhuis, G.W.: Gedragsproblemen bij 100 driejarigen, *Tijdschrift voor Jeugdgezondheidszorg* 15 (1983) 21–24.

Verhulst, F.C.: Psychische gezondheid bij Nederlandse kinderen, *Nederlands Tijdschrift voor Geneeskunde* 130 (1986) 2036–2040.

10 Health education

Informing parents about all aspects of the development and health of children is an essential part of the work of pre-school Child Health Care. Indeed information is pre-eminently a method to 'advance parental understanding of the health condition and (potential) development of their child and to increase their competence (health promoting behaviour)' (see Chapter 1). Even though health education has a long history, especially in pre-school Child Health Care (information on healthy nutrition, baby and child care and hygiene was one of the most important weapons against infant mortality), it is only in the last 20 years that the methods have been given scientific attention. Nowadays health education is interpreted as: 'all activities aimed at influencing the target group's attitudes and behaviour in the desired direction by means of communication' (Kok 1991).

Health education can only fractionally be distinguished as a separate activity within pre-school Child Health Care. The bulk of the information after all is given during the regular contacts between clinical team and parent. Generally, this is so-called anticipatory information; that is information on the physical and psychosocial development to be expected, anticipating the questions and problems that may arise as a result. Such information may in principle concern all subjects that are relevant in the context of child health and the development of the child or the parent-child relationship: care, nutrition, safety, growth, maturing, development, sensory organs, disturbances in development, education and so on. Information is also given about the various examinations carried out at the clinic. Parents are informed about immunizations, about screening, about the periodic health examination. This is usually done implicitly, that is to say during the dialogue between clinical medical officer or district nurse and parents around a specific action, as for instance the conducting of items of the Van Wiechen check-list[1]. Since the content of health education as well as the form in which it is given are to a high degree determined by the individual needs of the parents and the specific characteristics of the

---

[1]Partly based on the Denver Developmental Scale, the Van Wiechen check-list was developed in the early 1980s to promote the systematic examination of development (motor development, language and speech, personality and social behaviour) and to achieve uniform national registration. For details see Chapter 6, section 5.

individual child, formalization, although highly desirable, is extremely difficult. Its success moreover, is highly dependent on the measure in which there is a confidential relationship between the parent and the professional.

Health education that is concerned with individual parent and child characteristics must therefore of necessity be considered prevention to measure. In previous chapters we have pointed out the problems this entails for outcome assessment: it is practically impossible to assess results on the basis of criteria formulated in terms of objective 'gain in health'. This is not a matter of an unequivocal, once-only intervention, but rather a matter of recurring subjects of conversation. This makes it difficult to ascertain the time gap between the moment of information transfer and the moment at which outcome could be ascertained. Moreover, the subjects concerned are often treated in other places and at other points of time (by the media for instance). Next to this individually keyed education however, information activities of a more standardized character also take place within pre-school Child Health Care. Aspects are concerned that lend themselves to a population-directed approach: general information on growth and development and child-raising (the Growth Book, toddler information leaflets[2]), information relating to PKU/CHT screening (brochures), information on nutrition, safety (the Accident Prevention Cards[3]) and dental care.

Health education for the benefit of young people does not, of course, occur only within pre-school Child Health Care. Health Care for 4–19-year-olds has an explicit task here as well. To date, coordination between the two services has been insufficient.

As stated above, health education has developed extensively in the last few years. Several scientific institutes are developing models that can systematically handle the content, methods and outcome measurement of Health Education (De Haes 1983, Schuurman 1983, Rogmans 1984, Kok 1991). The application of such systems within pre-school Child Health Care however is still in its infancy. This is why in this chapter we present a model for the systematic set-up, implementation and evaluation of health

---

[2]The Growth Book has been issued to all parents of new-born babies in the Netherlands since 1978. It aims to give parents the information to help them care for and raise their children. For further details see section 10.1.2. Toddler information leaflets are folders with age-specific information on the development of the child. Subjects include: eating, sleeping, play, behaviour, toilet training, obstinacy.

[3]Accident Prevention Cards are a tool to promote safety, accidents being the major cause of death of children. Each card contains safety information aimed at a specific age group. They are handed out at child health clinics to make parents aware of accident risks at specific stages of the child's development. This helps parents to take safety measures in time.

education which seems to us very workable within the framework of pre-school Child Health Care. Systematic application of such a model could result in further development of standardized information in this field. However, we start this chapter with a survey of educational programmes that have been used in pre-school Child Health Care for some time and for which outcome data are known to a greater or lesser degree.

10.1 Investigation into the effectiveness of health education

In the Netherlands, few outcome studies are known with regard to education in fields important for pre-school Child Health Care (such as nutrition, dental care and accident prevention), according to several authors in the most recent survey of literature on the effectiveness of health education (Jonkers et al. 1988). The majority of the available data are on accident prevention, so that this subject will be treated more fully than the others.

10.1.1 Education on nutrition

In view of its primary preventive nature, information on nutrition has always been an important task of pre-school Child Health Care. To determine the content of the information, there must first be an understanding of the epidemiological relations between nutrition and health[4]. In the past, lack of clarity about these relationships often hampered effective education on nutrition. An example is the information on infant feeding. It appeared in practice that parents received diverse advice, depending on the clinic they attended and the person who gave the advice (Van der Avert 1986). In 1983, criticism occasioned the setting up of a study group that was commissioned to draw up general principles for the nutrition of healthy full-term babies in their first year of life. In 1985, the first edition was published of a literature search commissioned by this study group (Uitentuis 1985), supplemented by practical experience from the study group members. Since 1987, the study group has been testing these general principles against up-to-date scientific opinion (adjusting them where necessary) and has supplemented them with principles in the areas of alternative nutrition; nutrition in case of suspected food allergy; dietary

---

[4]For instance the interrelationship of dietary habits and the risk of cardiovascular disease, obesity, growth and development and food allergies.

advice for minor health disorders such as diarrhoea, vomiting, constipation and intestinal colic; vitamin K, follow-on formula feeds and supplementary vitamin A. In 1991, this new version was published as a bulletin from the Chief Medical Inspector: *Zuigelingenvoeding. Uitgangspunten en praktische aanbevelingen* (Infant feeding. Principles and practical recommendations). The principles are emphatically not to be taken as strict directions, but should serve as a basis for drawing up individual advice. 'The ultimate individual dietary advice mainly has to do with:

- recommended quantities of energy and nutrients
- parental preference
- weight/growth (growth chart)
- psychomotor development.

This principle means that different nutritional advice may be given to two children of the same age. It is essential that parents are consulted when formulating nutritional advice and that attention is paid to any particulars. It is therefore the professional's task to support the parents in their concern for their child's optimum nutrition' (Bulletin Chief Medical Inspector; see: GHI-bulletin 1991).

It is not clear, however, far these principles have met the criticism expressed by Van der Avert. The practical use of the new version is still to be evaluated.

10.1.2 The Growth Book: information on child care and child raising

The Growth Book is issued to all parents of new-born children in the Netherlands[5,6]. The booklet was first published in 1978 (5000 copies); by 1983 the annual issue was 200,000 copies and this number was maintained in subsequent years. Voorhoeve (1991) characterizes the Growth Book as a national document and a bestseller. For each new issue of the Growth Book the contents are adapted as necessary. 'As a result of remarks from users which the editors received through district nurses and clinical medical officers, adaptations were made in every reprint (Voorhoeve 1991). In the

---

[5]The publication of the Growth Book is financed out of the Special Medical Expenses Act (AWBZ).

[6]The Growth Book is available in several languages including English, Turkish, Moroccan and Chinese.

latest issue of the Growth Book, growth charts were included for the first time.

Hopman et al. (1992) investigated the contents of this national information medium and the degree to which the contents are based on scientific knowledge and social needs, concentrating on the teaching content of the Growth Book. They analysed the contents of the Growth Book for this aspect and sounded out the opinions of 183 parents of under-fives on the value of the Growth Book. 'The results were extremely clear.' the investigators state, 'the Growth Book appears to be unequalled as an information medium – the whole target group have the Growth Book, use it and actually understand its contents – but the contents gave them little satisfaction. It appears that the parents of toddlers are not able to find nearly enough child raising information in the Growth Book. The information it does contain, does not always satisfy their needs. Moreover, it does not keep up with current social developments and new scientific opinion' (Hopman & Vroonhof 1992). The investigators argue in favour of better utilization of the possibilities of the Growth Book as an information medium. Present conditions are optimal for this. The investigation shows that the Growth Book fulfils a number of functions for the parents: they use it as a baby book (they record events in it as well as the baby's development), it serves administrative purposes (parents apparently use the Growth Book as a file and safekeeping for all papers concerning the child and the clinic), has a reminder function (parents make notes in it on such things as nutritional advice and weight), is a source of information (parents use it as a reference book) and finally the Growth Book also has a communicative function (it provides parents with an incentive for talking to clinical staff).

It was assumed when preparing the first edition that the Growth Book should contain 50% guidance on child care and 50% guidance on upbringing. Hopman and Vroonhof however, find that the quantity of child rearing guidance does not meet this aim. Moreover they argue that the information is included in the Growth Book in the form of advice, which is outdated from the point of view of modern information science. They contend that the parents, being primarily responsible for their child, are quite capable of making their own choices about what to do, provided they are well-informed. Finally the guidance is found to be in disagreement with new scientific opinion and current social developments. The writers give three examples.

- The Growth Book states that a baby should preferably not be cared for by more than two or three adults; not only is this advice scientifically disputed (Van zerdoorn 1988 quoted in Hopman & Vroonhof 1992), but it is no longer socially acceptable (more and more often both parents remain in employment after the birth).

- The Growth Book emphasizes breast feeding, especially in view of the bonding of mother and child. 'Research however, shows that the quality of the bonding is not dependent on care...but on the carer's sensitivity for signals from the child' (Hopman & Vroonhof 1992).

- Watching television just before bedtime is advised against in the Growth Book; in reality watching *Sesame Street* is part of the going to bed ritual in many Dutch families.

Some advice is out-of-date, some ignores social developments and some does not link up with present-day parental needs. In conclusion, the writers say that, even though the content of the Growth Book does not meet current scientific and social demands, its educational possibilities are unique. The contents, according to the writers, should be adapted to new scientific views (both as to content and in the field of information science) and to new social developments and parents' needs.

A more or less concurring plea comes from Merkx (1992) and concerns a Personal Health Record for Child Health Care from birth to 19 years (analogous to the personal health records already developed in France, New Zealand and the United Kingdom); the main characteristic of such a record is that it is held by the parents. Merkx is of the opinion that a transformation of the present Growth Book in this direction would be the obvious course.

Advantages of such a record according to Merkx are:

- improved continuity of care (the transfer of data from the Community Health Care to the Municipal Health Services

- permanent availability of information to all medical care levels

- increased parental understanding of the information on their child's growth and development

- solution of the privacy problem: parents themselves can decide with whom they want to share specific information regarding their child

- greater parental involvement in the preventive care of their children.

With regard to the informative function the personal health record may fulfil an important additional role compared with the present Growth Book. The information in the present Growth Book is retained (after the necessary adaptation), but in addition the personal health record gives insight into the substance of care: for what and when is the child examined and what are the findings. Merkx however, also thinks the personal health record could have drawbacks: firstly, in the hands of parents the record could often be lost; secondly, recording sensitive information becomes more difficult and parents could get worried unnecessarily or misinterpret the information. As to the first objection, Merkx states that the experience with the Growth Book is that the percentage of lost copies is low. Hopman and Vroonhof (1992) arrive at the same result: the 183 parents polled by them kept the Growth Book carefully. With regard to the second objection, Merkx poses that openness on sensitive subjects (for instance suspected child abuse) may assist early detection. Moreover, experts will always have the option of making notes outside the personal health record in the regular medical record (which will be retained). Research in the United Kingdom among doctors and nurses did not confirm the second objection[7].

10.1.3 Dental health education

For a number of reasons, dental health education has a special place within health education. It is one of the first fields in which large scale information activities were held. The evaluation research available on these activities however, is mainly of an exploratory and descriptive nature; the number of thorough outcome studies is small (Saan 1988). Dental health education aims at preventing dental decay and crooked teeth. Information is the means of trying to influence knowledge, attitude and behaviour with reference to brushing teeth, regular visits to the dentist, sweets, use of fluoride (prevention of caries) and thumb and finger sucking (prevention of deviant tooth positions). The first projects in this field in the Netherlands were set up in the late 1960s and were notably targeted at reduction of the high incidence of caries (at that time).

Evaluation of the projects proved them to have effected a reduction in caries, which however was put in perspective because in a later phase of evaluation a general reduction in caries was shown to have taken place in the Netherlands. It appears from a literature search by Saan (1988) that measures such as the availability of fluoride in toothpastes and the use of these toothpastes, as well as changes in the patterns of nutrition and visits to the dentist, play a considerable part in the final effects of dental health education (Saan 1988). Kalsbeek & Verrips (1991), on the basis of an investigation into the long-term effects of preventive dental care for toddlers in Tiel, arrive at a somewhat different conclusion, namely that the mother's motivation for caries prevention (ascertained when the child is aged 2 years) appears to have a considerable influence on the caries

---

[7]Unfortunately it was not clear from the text of the article concerned which study this was.

experience[8] of the child at ages 6 and 15 years. No caries preventive outcome of professional dental care from an early age or of the use of fluoride tablets could be demonstrated. For dental health in the long term it appears to be essential that the mother begins looking after her child's teeth at an early age (Kalsbeek & Verrips 1991).

10.1.4 Accident prevention

Every year accidents claim more children's lives than the six major childhood diseases taken together (Rogmans 1984, De Leeuw 1988). In regard to morbidity as a result of accidents pre-school children are a major high-risk group too. In the past 10 years increasing attention has been paid to the prevention of accidents involving young children; the 2000 Memorandum (Ministry of Welfare, Health and Cultural Affairs 1986) gives high priority to the pre-school age group. Accidents can be prevented by means of passive prevention (making the environment safer[9]), as well as by active prevention (endeavouring to influence parental behaviour that affects the safety of the environment). The emphasis in accident prevention is now on safety education. Important conditions for the development of educational programmes are understanding the nature and extent of the problem and understanding the behavioural determinants[10]. Accident research, especially as regards accidents other than traffic and industrial accidents made a slow start in the Netherlands (Rogmans 1984, De Leeuw 1988). According to Rogmans (1984) one of the major causes is to be found in methodological problems, such as the lack of an unequivocal definition, the relative rarity of accidents, their complexity and the problem of the *ex-postfacto* testimony.

10.1.4.1 The size of the problem

Epidemiological understanding of the magnitude and nature of accidents involving young children is a prime requirement for the development of prevention programmes. There has been insight into mortality as a result of accidents for a long time. Registration of fatal accidents is performed by the Central Bureau of Statistics (Register of causes of death). However, insight into morbidity (as far as professional help is called in) is only of recent date.

---

[8]The caries experience is expressed by the total of the numbers of untreated caries lesions, fillings and extractions (Kalsbeek & Verrips 1991).

[9]Much has already been done in this field. Think of child-resistant containers, safe toys, safe children's nightwear and such.

[10]Recently such a problem analysis was made on burns to young children (Van Rijn et al. 1989, 1990, Van Rijn 1991).

The Foundation for Consumer and Safety (Stichting Consument en Veiligheid, SCV) has initiated a system of registration to this end, called PORS (domestic accidents registration). PORS has been operative since 1983. Records are kept of all domestic accidents in the casualty departments of 14 hospitals in the Netherlands. Another registration system which is important in this respect is the National Medical Registration (Landelijke Medische Registratie LMR) conducted by the Health Care Information Institution (Stichting Informatievoorziening Gezondheidszorg SIG); this institution registers the use of intramural health care in hospitals.

Mortality from accidents involving children has dropped considerably in the past few years. De Jonge (1991) draws this conclusion from the CBS registration of death by accidents in the 1979 to 1989 period. For the population of children (birth to 4 years) there was a drop of some 50%. In 1979, the number of children killed in accidents (including traffic accidents and drowning, as well as domestic accidents) was 908 per 1,000,000 children from birth to 4 years. In 1989, this number was 457 per 1,000,000 children from birth to 4 years. There is an especially spectacular drop with regard to drowning (children of one to 4 years) and suffocation (children from birth to 1 year). Such a drop however, is not seen in all areas: the increased number of fatal traffic accidents in which babies are involved is striking (22:1,000,000 in 1979 to 53:1,000,000 in 1989). Further analysis of the data of a number of consecutive years is required to decide if the above comparison indicates a trend.

Such a trend analysis, of the data gathered by PORS (Schoots & Mulder 1991), was published for the first time in 1991 by the Foundation for Consumer and Safety. The percentage of accidents involving children up to the age of 4 years was seen to decrease by 11% in the 1984–1989 period. This is a gratifying development. In regard to the above mentioned trend analysis, Rogmans (1991) suggests that the trend indications must not be seen as real drops in incidence, nor does this first analysis allow conclusions with reference to the outcome of preventive interventions. Other developments play a part in the drop in the number of accidents as well: 'Generally we may assume that with a continuing increase in prosperity there will be an increase in the possibilities (for instance the general level of education), in the means (share of spendable income made available for a higher safety level of products and amenities purchased) and the level of community facilities (safety level of play areas, social housing, environment and so on). This should lead to a process of declining accident figures, notably of the very serious, fatal injuries, for instance a fall from a high building, drowning, and burns from an open fire. Moreover, better casualty services and medical treatment may well have reduced mortality' (Rogmans 1991). Health education, provided it is developed well, has a high potential for further reducing the number of accidents involving young children.

10.1.4.2 Education in the clinic on accident prevention

The aim of accident prevention education in the clinic is to motivate parents to adopt safety conscious behaviour (Rogmans 1984). Safety conscious behaviour means taking preventive measures that make the environment in which the child grows up safer in a direct way. Influencing behaviour by increasing the knowledge and changing the attitudes of parents is the core of accident prevention. Various studies have shown that parents have insufficient insight into the relationship between the normal development of children and the attendant risks of accidents (Rivara & Howard 1982, Rogmans 1984, Wortel & Ooyendijk 1988). In 1984 and 1985, the Foundation for Consumer and Safety, in cooperation with the then National Cross Association[11] and the Institute for Information on Education and Play (Stichting Spel-en Opvoedingsvoorlichting) developed written information for individual accident prevention in pre-school Child Health Care.

A number of evaluation studies were carried out on the education given in clinics on accident prevention (among others by Stompedissel et al. 1989, De Geus 1990). The research that De Geus was commissioned to do by the Foundation for Consumer and Safety concerned a process evaluation of education on accident prevention, as given in nine out of the total of 15 regions corresponding with the areas of the member institutions of the National Association for Community Nursing and Home Care. In the main, this process evaluation may be considered representative for the situation nationwide. Broadly speaking, the findings of De Geus correspond to the results of the research by Stompedissel et al. (1989); this research was done in five clinics in Rotterdam and deals with the use of and opinions on Accident Prevention Cards.

Conclusions drawn from the research data by De Geus are:

- Information on child safety is inadequately underpinned with respect to theory and information science: specific targets are lacking, ways to influence parental attitude and behaviour have been insufficiently worked out.

---

[11]For a long time Cross Associations (Kruisverenigingen) have been active in the Netherlands in the fields of social and preventive medicine and home nursing on behalf of their members as well as of the general public. The National Cross Association (Nationale Kruisvereniging) represented the regional cross associations at national level. In 1990, the National Cross Association merged with the National Council for Home Help (Centrale Raad voor de Gezinsverzorging) to form the National Association for Community Nursing and Home Care (Landelijke Vereniging voor Thuiszorg), established at Bunnik. In this book the regional organizations will be referred to as Community Health Care.

- Individual education, targeted at influencing attitudes, has hardly taken shape. Partly as a result, the printed material functions as an aim in itself rather than as a (supportive) means.

- Individual education does not adequately live up to its promise. This partly results from objective factors such as lack of money and heavy work loads and partly from individual factors such as motivation, knowledge and skills.

The following recommendations are made:

- to formulate a well defined framework (prevention policy, under-pinning consistent with information science, targets) within which education on accident prevention in the clinics should take place

- to maintain the Child Health Clinic channel because of the potentially vast range

- to remove as many impediments as possible in methods of giving information: increasing the time available for a visit; specific extra training of clinical staff; adaptation of the methods of working with the information material.

Process assessments may offer significant points of departure for modifications of education practice. The recommendations by De Geus could give direction to this. What is lacking in the field of accident prevention is thorough outcome assessment (De Leeuw 1988). Some outcome studies in this field have been done in other countries, but according to De Leeuw these are characterized by less effective research designs (no or non-equivalent control groups or the use of lower level outcome measures); because of these shortcomings failure or success cannot be ascribed unequivocally to the quality of the information programme.

10.2 A model for the systematic setting up, implementation and assessment of health education

In the above, some examples of standardized programmed prevention in the field of health education have been discussed. Consideration of these examples reveals some unanswered questions: how are priorities to be set (which are the major health problems on which education is necessary and possible), how are information programmes to be developed and how are such programmes to be assessed? At the request of the Working Party, the

Department of Health Education of Limburg State University has presented a general model for the systematic setting up, implementing and assessing of health education. Such a model is not only important with a view to new activities in the field of health eduction, it may also serve as a frame of reference in assessing existing educational activities. Priorities for health education should be set on the basis of the formula 'importance multiplied by susceptibility': the problems and behaviour to be given top priority must first be decided upon on the basis of epidemiological research, then the extent should be ascertained to which this behaviour could be influenced by education, combined with facilities and possibly regulation. An intervention developed in this way should be tested in a trial project and systematically assessed both as to process and to outcome. Interventions that prove successful may subsequently be introduced on a large scale.

In the first instance, such planned setting up and assessment of education interventions will require a relatively large investment, entailing various forms of research: epidemiological research, research into determinants, development of the intervention, assessment research. The planning stage begins by determining the seriousness and size of the problem. Subsequently, an analysis has to be made of what behaviour is related to the problem and whose behaviour this is. Finally the determinants of the behaviour have to be investigated. To be able to influence behaviour it is necessary to understand the reasons people have for specific behaviour. Socio-psychologists distinguish three types of behaviour determinants: attitude, social influence and self-effectiveness (the ASE model: Kok & Green 1990) (Figure 1).

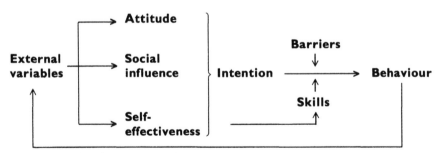

Figure 1 Model of behavioural determinants.

According to the model in Figure 1, attitude, social standards and self-effectiveness predict intention. Intention then predicts behaviour. External (outside the model) variables, such as demographic factors, are supposed to influence behaviour only through the three determinants and the intention. It is moreover, indicated in the model that there may be barriers present between intention and behaviour and that skills to exhibit the behaviour may be lacking. In itself, intention is a good predictor of the actual behaviour, but the theory also indicates that self-effectiveness is the assessment of the skills needed and (perhaps owing to that) the possibility to overcome barriers. When, finally, somebody exhibits the behaviour or tries to do so, this will induce feedback by which in turn the determinants are influenced. Attitude is the weighing up of all pros and cons of the behaviour, not therefore only the health or safety considerations, but also aspects such as expensive, bothersome, inconvenient, conflicting with standards and values, and so on. Social influence may be direct or indirect: direct in so far as others expect specific behaviour, indirect if others exhibit that behaviour (modelling). Self-effectiveness is the person's assessment of his or her ability to exhibit the behaviour. Behaviour determinants are diverse and sometimes complex. Nevertheless, understanding of determinants is necessary to develop interventions. There are too many instances already of interventions targeted (with hindsight) on the wrong behaviour determinants. This is wasteful and may be counterproductive (Kok & Green 1990).

On the basis of these three stages, an intervention to guide behaviour can be developed. Education is one possibility for this. Kok argues for considering health education within the greater whole of a health promotion policy. Other options to influence behaviour are: regulation (making behaviour mandatory or forbidding it, together with the necessary sanctions/monitoring) or measures to facilitate the desired behaviour.

	Message	Recipient	Channel	Source	Measures
Attention and understanding					
Change in determinants and behaviour					
Maintaining behaviour change					

Figure 2 Model of behaviour change by education.

The development of programmes for change in behaviour by education can be presented in a matrix (Figure 2). Briefly, this model amounts to the following: firstly communication must be effected between messenger and recipient; secondly changes in behaviour must take place and finally habit forming of the changed behaviour should be sought. Once-only changes of behaviour do not (usually) suffice[12]. The last phase is the assessment. This investigation provides information on the correctness of all decisions taken during the planning procedure and therefore gives indications for

---

[12]For an elaboration of the model see Van Rijn (1991) and McGuire (1985).

improvements in the intervention. A distinction should be made here between outcome assessment and process assessment. Outcome assessment investigates whether the object in view has been reached, namely a reduction in the problem found at the beginning of the planning stage. Process assessment investigates whether the intermediate steps have been taken as intended, such as implementation, carrying out of intervention, and changes in the behaviour determinants. If the aim of the education has not been achieved, the results of the assessment provide indications for the reasons for this failure. Outcome assessment cannot yield meaningful information if the elementary methodological principles are not observed (Jonkers et al. 1988): notably the use of pre- and post-measurements and the use of a control group. The change seen in the experimental group is compared with the same difference in the control group that was not given the intervention. Only then can a pronouncement be made on the effectiveness, if any, of the intervention in the experimental group. Often post-verification is required in the longer term, because the outcome of intervention is sometimes quickly lost, whereas we are, on the contrary, interested in lasting outcome. The above shows that it is difficult to assess national interventions because of the absence of a control group. In this instance, it is essential to have several pre-measurements over a longer period, so that a base-line is known. Then an intervention may be considered effective if the outcome deviates from the base-line. The final criterion is whether the problem has been reduced, but in practice other outcome measures are often used, for instance identifying changed behaviour in the target group. Such an intermediate outcome measure as a test for success can only be justified if the relationship between behaviour and problem is obvious. If the assessment stage proves the intervention to be effective, it will have to be implemented on a large scale. This is an activity with its own potential and difficulties.

10.3 Conclusions

Health education is a major aspect of pre-school Child Health Care. From the historical point of view, education has been one of the more important means since the founding of Child Health Clinics and has probably contributed to a considerable degree to improved public health. The practice established through the years however is still poorly standardized at present. It lacks a system for:

- setting priorities for health problems (it should be noted that priorities can or must be established at different levels: national, regional and local; it is important that health profiles of the groups to be distinguished are available at these different levels)

- developing programmes for health education
- assessing present and future education programmes.

10.4 Recommendations

- It is recommended that priorities be established among the major issues and problems in which health education can play a part. Priorities should be set on the basis of *inter alia* epidemiological data, problem analysis and research into determinants, after investigation of the feasibility of prevention by means of influencing behaviour. Subsequently interventions have to be developed for the problems mentioned, to be implemented in a test area and to be assessed (in a methodologically correct manner). The model described in section 10.2 could be used for such a system.

- It is recommended that the information methods now in practical use in pre-school Child Health Care be assessed as far as possible, in accordance with the model mentioned in section 10.1. This applies in any case to educational methods that are to be newly introduced.

- In case of further assessment of the Growth Book, attention should be paid not only to the content of the book as a means of information, but also the interrelationship should be established with the possible development of a personal health record.

- Further gearing should take place of health education offered within the framework of pre-school Child Health Care and what is offered in other sectors, notably Child Health Care for 4–19-year-olds.

References

Avert, F.J. van der: Introductie nieuwe uitgangspunten zuigelingenvoeding, *Voeding* 47 (1986) 81–84.

Geus, G.H. de: *Voorlichting over Kinderveiligheid op Consultatiebureaus. Evaluatie-onderzoek van de voorlichtingspraktijk*, Amsterdam: Stichting Consument en Veiligheid, 1990.

Haes, W.F.M. de: *Gedragswetenschappelijk onderzoek ten dienste van gezondheidsvoorlichting enopvoeding*, Lisse 1983.

Hopman, M.J.G. & Vroonhof, C.E.M.: Ouders van een- tot vierjarigen zoeken vergeefs antwoord op opvoedingsvragen, *Maatschappelijke Gezondheidszorg* 20 jan/febr (1992) 34–37.

Jonge, G.A. de: Veiligheid (0–19 jaar) in 10 jaar sterk verbeterd!, *Tijdschrift voor Jeugdgezondheidszorg* 23 (1991) 4, 50–54.

Jonkers, R., Haes, W.F.M. de, Kok, G.J., Liedekerken, P.C., Saan, J.A.M.: *Effectiviteit van Gezondheidsvoorlichting enopvoeding*, Utrecht 1988.

Kalsbeek, H., Verrips, G.H.: *Lange-termijn-effecten van preventieve tandzorg bij kleuters*, Leiden: NIPG/TNO, 1991.

Kok, G.J. & Green, L.W.: Onderzoek ter ondersteuning van de GVO-praktijk: een pleidooi voor meer samenwerking, *Tijdschrift Gezondheidsbevordering* 11 (1990) 5–12.

Kok, G.J.: *Jeugdgezondheidszorg en gezondheidsvoorlichting (GVO)*, interne publikatie Project Integrale Evaluatie Jeugdgezondheidszorg, Utrecht: Rijksuniversiteit Utrecht, 1991.

Leeuw, E. de: De effectiviteit van voorlichting ter voorkoming van ongevallen in de privésfeer, in: Jonkers, R. et al. (red.): *Effectiviteit van Gezondheidsvoorlichting enopvoeding*, Utrecht 1988, pp.254-260.

McGuire, W.J.: Attitudes and attitude changes, in: Lindsay, G. & Aronson, E. (eds.): *Handbook of Social Psychology: Volume II*, New York 1985.

Merkx, J.A.M.: Pleidooi voor een Persoonlijk Gezondheidsdossier, *Maatschappelijke Gezondheidszorg* 20 January/February (1992) 24–26.

Ministerie van WVC: *Over de ontwikkeling van gezondheidsbeleid: feiten, beschouwingen en beleidsvoornemens (Nota 2000)*, Den Haag: Sdu Uitgeverij, 1986.

Rijn, O. van, Bouter, L.M., Meertens, R.M., Grol, M.E.C., Kok, G.J., Mulder, S.: *Brandwonden bij 0–4 jarige kinderen. Verslag van een etiologisch patiënt-controle-onderzoek*, Amsterdam: Stichting Consument en Veiligheid, 1989.

Rijn, O.J.L., Meertens, R.M., Bouter, L.M., Grol, M.E.C., Kok, G.J.: *Determinanten van veiligheidsgedrag van ouders ter preventie van brandwonden bij 0–4 jarige kinderen. Een exploratieve studie*, Amsterdam: Stichting Consument en Veiligheid, 1990.

Rijn, O.J.L.: *Burn injuries among young children. Incidence, aetiology and determinants of behavioural risk factors*, Maastricht 1991 (dissertation).

Rivara, S.P. & Howard, D.: Parental knowledge of child development and injury risks. *Journal of Development and Behavioural Pediatrics* 3 (1982), p. 2.

Rogmans, W.H.J.: *Jonge kinderen en ongevalsrisico's buiten het verkeer*, Leiden 1984 (dissertation).

Rogmans, W.H.J.: Trends in letsels door ongevallan in de privésfeer. *Tijdschrift voor Jeugdgezondheidszorg* 23 (1991) 5, p.76.

Saan, J.A.M.: De effectiviteit van TGVO, in: Jonkers, R. et al. (red.): *Effectiviteit van Gezondheidsvoorlichting enopvoeding*, Utrecht 1988, pp.191–198.

Schoots, W. & Mulder, S.: *Trends in privé-ongevallen 1984–1988. Resultaten van trendanalyses, uitgevoerd op gegevens van het Privé Ongevallen Registratie Systeem*, Amsterdam: Stichting Consument en Veiligheid, 1991.

Schuurman, J.H.: *Gezondheidsvoorlichting enopvoeding; onderzoek en aktie met betrekking tot harten vaatziekten, geslachtsziekten en roken*, Lisse 1983.

Stompedissel, I., Wortel, E., Groen in 't Woud, G.W.M.: Veiligheidskaarten – Gebruik en opvattingen, *Tijdschrift voor Jeugdgezondheidszorg* 21 (1989) 5, 73–75.

Uitentuis, J.: Zuigelingenvoeding, de huidige inzichten, *Tijdschrift voor Kindergeneeskunde* 53 (1985) suppl. 1–48.

Voorhoeve, H.W.A.: 14e druk Groeiboek, *Tijdschrift voor Jeugdgezondheidszorg* 23 (1991) 6, 96.

Wortel, E. & Oijendijk, W.T.M.: *Preventie van privéongevallen bij kinderen: onderzoek naar preventief gedrag bij onders en gedragsdeterminanten*. Leiden: NIPG/TNO (1988).

Further reading

Assema, P. van, Hospers, H.J., Liedekerken, P.C.: De effectiviteit van voedingsvoorlichting, in: Jonkers, R. et al. (red.): *Effectiviteit van Gezondheids-voorlichting enopvoeding*, Utrecht 1988, pp.170–181.

Bakker, E.C. & Burg-Beijk, P.C. van de: *Veiligheidskaarten: wat betekenen ze voor onze kliënten? Een onderzoek naar de betekenis van de verstrekking van veiligheidskaarten aan ouders van kinderen van 0–4 jaar*, Kruisvereniging West Overijssel 1989.

Balledux, M., Mare, J. de, Winter, M. de: *Project Integrale Evaluatie Jeugdgezondheidszorg. Literatuurstudies*, Utrecht: Rijksuniversiteit Utrecht, 1991.

Bergink, A.H.: Dodelijke ongevallen bij kinderen in Den Haag in de periode 1986–1990, *Tijdschrift voor Jeugdgezondheidszorg* 23 (1991) 4, 58–60.

Boer, D.J. den, Kok, G., Hospers, H.J., Gerards, F.M. & Strecher, V.J.: Health education strategies for attributional retraining and self-efficacy improvement, *Health Education Research* 5 (1991).

Bouter, L.M., Rijn, O.J.L. van, Kok, G.: Importance of planned health education for burn injury prevention, *Burns* 16 (1990) 3, 198–202.

Burg-Beijk, P.C. van der: Veiligheidskaarten, een waardevol hulpmiddel. Verslag van een onderzoek, *Tijdschrift voor Jeugdgezondheidszorg* 22 (1990) 5, 67–68.

Damoiseaux, V., Gerards, F.M., Kok, G.J., Nijhuis, F. (red.): *Gezondheidsvoorlichting enopvoeding; van analyse tot effecten*, Assen/Maastricht 1987.

Emans, B.: Produkten procesevaluatie van GVO, *Gezondheid en maatschappij* 5 (1983) 200–206.

GHI-bulletin: *Zuigelingenvoeding. Uitgangspunten en praktische aanbevelingen*, Rijswijk 1991.

Kelly, B., Sein, C., McCarthy, P.L.: Safety education in a pediatric primary care setting, *Pediatrics* 79 (1987) 818–824.

Kok, G.J. & Jonkers-Kuiper, L. (red.): *Lokale gezondheidsinitiatieven*, Maastricht 1991.

Kuiper, C.M.: *Toepassing van richtlijnen voor de voeding van zuigelingen*, Leiden 1988.

Kuiper, C.M. & Mey-Kremers, A.J.M.: Voedingsrichtlijnen en zuigelingenconsultatie-bureaus, *Tijdschrift voor Jeugdgezondheidszorg* 22 (1990) 2, 26–29.

Laidman, P.: *Health visiting and preventing accidents to children*, Research Report no.12, Child Accident Prevention Trust, London 1987.

Peterson, L. & Mori, L.: Prevention of Child Injury: An overview of Targets, Methods and Tactics for Psychologists, *Journal of Consulting and Clinical Psychology* 53 (1985) 586–595.

Pless, I.B. & Arsenault, L.: The Role of Health Education in the Prevention of Injuries to Children, *Journal of Social Issues* 43 (1987) 87–103.

Quant, W. & Willemse, C.: Het consultatiebureau mag geen testbatterij worden, *Tijdschrift voor Gezondheid en Politiek* December (1990) 19–20.

Roberts, M.C., Elkins, P.D., Royal, G.P.: Psychological applications to the Prevention of Accidents and Illness, in: M.C.Roberts & L. Peterson (eds.): *Prevention of Problems in childhood: Psychological Research and Applications*, New York 1984, pp.173-199.

Walle-Sevenster, J. de & Kok, G.J.: *Gezondheidsbevordering en armoede*, Bleiswijk 1991.

11 Activities directed at the social and physical environment of children and parents

In Chapter 1 of this report the so-called ecological health model was chosen as the conceptual framework for pre-school Child Health Care. In the model, health and sickness are described as the product of four determinants: physical factors, health behaviour, the social and physical environment, and finally the care system. In this chapter the focus is on the social and physical environment of children and parents as a health determinant. It should be made clear that we are concerned with a very broad range of factors about which only extremely fragmentary scientific data are as yet available. So here we shall have to make do with a preliminary general description. It is clear that arrears in scientific research in this field will have to be made good. We first indicate which environmental factors may be relevant to the health and wellbeing of children and parents (section 11.1). Consideration is then given to the possibilities for preventive action on the part of pre-school Child Health Care (section 11.2). Finally several consequences for the methods employed by pre-school Child Health Care are outlined.

11.1 Health and environment factors

Today, illness, health, and normal or problematic development are generally seen against the background of a complex combination of personally or environmentally linked variables. In the medical world the term multi-causality is often used in this context; in the social sciences that specifically concern themselves with child development, the concept transactional development[1] is current. In both branches of science there has recently been renewed appreciation of the environment as a determinant of health and development. This appreciation is modern, but far from new. Pre-school health care, as the successor to social hygiene, has its historical roots in the relationship between health and environment. In their research into and their struggle against the very high infant and child

---

[1]See also Chapter 6: Developmental surveillance.

mortality in the last century, the social hygienists discovered that there was a clear relationship between health, health behaviour, and environmental factors. They demonstrated that social conditions such as poverty, bad working conditions, poor housing, undernourishment, and the absence of hygienic facilities (clean water, sewerage) were to a great extent responsible for the great differences in morbidity and mortality for each socio-economic class.

11.1.1 Social inequality

Although the general health condition of the population has improved considerably since the beginning of this century, owing in part to increased prosperity and to improved facilities, the philosophy of the hygienists has lost little topicality. After all, in the present day there is also every reason to view the health and development of children in the light of social relationships. Now too, there are still major socio-economic and socio-cultural differences in children's health and development chances (Municipal Health Service Amsterdam 1980, Scientific Council on National Policy; see: WRR 1987). Children from so-called deprived backgrounds score poorly on many health indicators; the prenatal and infant mortality in children from the weakest environments (measured by the father's occupation) is several times that of those from the strongest environments (Norbeck et al. 1983) and children from the poorest environments do far worse in characteristics such as birth weight and growth in length (see among others Nijhuis 1989).

Thus social inequality may be taken to be an important environmental determinant of children's health and wellbeing. On a material level, that is to say in the daily reality of parents and children, this inequality is manifested in, among other things, the material quality of primary living conditions (including housing, finances, safety) and the quality of the facilities (after-school care possibilities, education, play space in the neighbourhood). It will be evident that a culmination of such unfavourable conditions can also adversely influence the psycho-social and educational climate in the families concerned (Ministry of Welfare, Public Health and Cultural Affairs 1992). The ecology of the family (i.e. the specific situation and location) has, according to the psychologist Hermanns, a greater influence on development and upbringing than is generally assumed (Hermanns 1992). In this connection he refers to studies carried out by Rutter which show that children from inner cities display more behavioural problems and psychological problems than children from small towns and villages (Rutter 1978, 1981), and to overview studies by Bronfenbrenner which point to school problems and psychological and social problems in children from families hit by unemployment and low incomes (Bronfen-brenner 1986).

11.1.2 Physical environment

In addition to considering health determinants that are linked to the phenomenon of social inequality (that is to say determinants which especially concern children in socially deprived situations), account must be taken of environmental determinants which operate at the level of the entire population. Danger from traffic and lack of safe places for playing in the neighbourhood are examples. In addition, the health and wellbeing of children is being increasingly threatened by the deterioration of the physical environment. There are numerous indications that the diminishing quality of soil, air and water have and will have a negative effect on children's health.

11.1.3 Primary lifeworld

Children's primary lifeworld, the family, is a major source of socio-cultural influence on the health and wellbeing of, notably, young children. It is probably typical of the fast changes taking place within this sphere of influence that the term family life has itself become too restricted to describe the variety of arrangements within which children grow up. An important reason for describing such processes of change as socio-cultural determinants of health and wellbeing is that the factors concerned indeed affect the individual child and family, but at the same time go far beyond the individual level. In other words, we are concerned with health determinants which have a strong impact at population level. For a number of years now in the Netherlands, we have been familiar with a growing number of one-parent families, adoptive families, step-families, and cooperative houses where there are children. The effect that the emergence and existence of these new ways of living have on the health and development of children is still to a great extent unknown. What is known is that there is a greater chance of psycho-social problems, often as a result of a precarious socio-economic situation, within one-parent families and families involved in divorce proceedings. Moreover, it may be assumed that because of the decreasing number of children in each family, the parents will in any case be less experienced in bringing up and caring for children.

Not only has there been a great change in recent years in the composition of primary forms of living together, but mutual relationships have also changed. According to Van den Dungen the modern Western family has developed into a kind of greenhouse in which 'numerous stresses originate in a space that is practically closed off from the outside world' (Van den Dungen 1989). As a result of the strict separation between the inner world and the outside world, between the family and society, young children have become extremely subject to the family moods and tempers. One of the consequences can be that family secrets, such as mistreatment and sexual abuse, remain behind closed doors for a long time. As the individualization of family members intensifies (Brinkgreve & De Regt 1990), so the availability of social support outside the family becomes even more important. In a recent study on the determinants of mental health, Bosma and Hosman (1990) point to the protective character a social support network can have with regard to mental health.

11.1.4 Professionalization

The last socio-cultural environmental determinant to which attention should be drawn in this regard, is the (alleged) parental uncertainty on upbringing and the related professionalization of the primary lifeworld. The current cultural pattern of relations with children and of their upbringing is sometimes described as the helping mode, an expression of a highly developed psychological consciousness in relation to children, whereby the parental task is placed under a magnifying-glass (DeMause 1976). Where traditional frames of reference, such as religion and family traditions are gradually being eroded, a growing need for and supply of professional information and help is created. Besides the undoubtedly positive aspects, this professionalization of parenthood also has disadvantages. Liljeström (1983) considers the almost unlimited trust that parents in the Western world appear to place in science and professionalism, to be a demoralizing factor in the process of upbringing. Parents are in danger of becoming ever greater laymen in their own field, that of parenthood (De Winter 1986). This is important for pre-school Child Health Care; since specifically in the period when parents have young children they are confronted with numerous questions and uncertainties, whereby they may drift into a dependency relationship with professionals. So it is of even greater importance that pre-school Child Health Care explicitly emphasizes and stimulates parents' own competence and responsibility.

11.2 Implications for pre-school Child Health Care: recognition, guidance and cooperation

As outlined above, the health and development of young children display a notable degree of interrelationship with social, cultural and physical environmental factors. After a long period in which these environmental factors seemed to have faded into the background in the entire health care sector, a reappraisal of this relationship is gradually being made. One source of inspiration for this is the WHO programme *Health for All by the*

Year 2000, adapted for the Netherlands as *Nota 2000*. According to Nijhuis (1989) it is essential that pre-school Child Health Care is explicitly oriented to social circumstances which have relevance for health. In his view 'pre-school Child Health Care should give a prominent place to explicit social involvement', which 'means a rather essential new orientation in theory and practice, away from the traditional medical needs' and which demands 'explicit focusing on a healthy existence, also in the social sense' from health professionals. A similar point of view is expressed by De Winter (1990): A pre-school Child Health Care service that concerns itself with the 'quality of childhood existence' must satisfy three requirements: besides the provision of effective individual preventive health care for all children; and the provision of personal support and care to the parents and children who need them; Child Health Care must also promote social care at the system level.

Therefore, in its concern for health and wellbeing, pre-school Child Health Care should aim, by recognition and guidance, at structural factors which are (in part) at the roots of the problems of individual parents and children. Moreover, such a view means that pre-school Child Health Care should maintain well-defined forms of cooperation with agencies that are concerned with child day-care, education, social welfare planning, urban and traffic planning. In *Nota 2000* this is described as facet policy. On the basis of its specific expertise pre-school Child Health Care, in its qualities of identifying and advising, can function in relation to such social sectors which may be assumed to have a relevant influence on certain health determinants. Since the pre-school health service's major domain is at local level, recognition and guidance should be specifically aimed at this level. A possible consequence of this social orientation is that special attention must be given to groups of parents and children that are particularly vulnerable to health and social welfare problems, due to a culmination of unfavourable environmental determinants (Ministry of Welfare, Public Health and Cultural Affairs 1992). Several examples of such a method of working can already be found in practice, both within the pre-school Child Health Care service and between this service and other organizations. For instance in the Amsterdam Child Health Care this way of working has already been outlined in a policy plan (Municipal Health Service Amsterdam; see: GG & GD Amsterdam 1990).

In a number of places pre-school Child Health Care already participates in child welfare service community networks. These networks, in which agencies for day-care, education and child welfare are represented, concern themselves specifically with problems in deprived neighbourhoods. They aim at early recognition of and intervention in problem situations at an individual level, as well as at social identification (Geelen et al. 1989, Wilbrink-Griffioen & Van Eyck 1990). Nijhuis calls population participation the most important basic principle for a socially oriented Child Health

Care. This dialogue is needed for two reasons, firstly to be able to establish the child's problems that need attention and secondly to create a basis for realizing adequate measures or for enlarging health consciousness (Nijhuis 1989). As put forward earlier, to avoid too great a dependence on the professional system, the responsibility of (groups of) parents should be the starting point of a Child Health Care policy. There are already a number of examples of such active involvement of parents. In many municipalities, improvements in the home environment are brought about in a dialogue with parents, for instance those regarding safe playgrounds and traffic situations. It seems superfluous to state that the areas of attention mentioned here are not exclusively tasks of pre-school Child Health Care. In fact dialogue and cooperation with other relevant sectors in society will be the rule rather than the exception. For the pre-school Child Health Care service, this social orientation means a continual analysis of factors and phenomena which may threaten, but also promote, the quality of life in terms of health and wellbeing. Child health professionals have to be actively engaged in this analysis and they must identify and advise in regard to health facets, such as environmental policy, urban and community planning, social welfare policy and education. The reverse also applies: the neighbourhood, the day-care centre, the city council should be able to influence Child Health Care policy by means of the information they provide.

A final important item is the careful registration of health threatening risk factors. An example is the *Atlas of Young Almere* in which a profile is sketched of the young people in Almere (a new town in the Netherlands), on the basis of integrated data on demography, education, socio-cultural facilities, housing, employment, health services and social services (Project Group Integrated Youth Policy Almere/Project Group Healthy Flevoland Towns; see: Projectgroep geïntegreerd jeugdbeleid 1992).

11.3 Consequences for policy, professionals and executive organizations

Being based on an ecological health model, pre-school Child Health Care cannot ignore the relevant influences from their social and physical environment on the health and wellbeing of parents and children. This is by no means to say that doctors and district nurses working in this field have no attention or eye for such a line of approach. However, the problem is that activities in this direction are not as yet a structural part of their duties and therefore often take place on an *ad hoc* basis. Structural embedding of such a perspective will mean an expansion of the interpretation of the task of present pre-school Child Health Care or, in other words, a re-assessment of the original points of departure and working methods on which its founding and social embedding were based. Naturally today's working methods should be adapted to changed social conditions, state of health, health needs and scientific insights. Supported by an insight into the health needs of parents and children, and in cooperation with other social agencies and organizations, pre-school Child Health Care can develop along these lines into what Nijhuis calls 'a consultant on matters of social decision-making and on the expansion of insight into health needs, as an advocate of health affairs' (Nijhuis 1989).

It will be clear that the point of view described here needs to be further consolidated and made operational. Systematically and actively influencing socio-cultural and physical circumstances that are relevant for the health and wellbeing of young children, demands a change in attitude from agencies responsible for policy, executive organizations and professionals in pre-school Child Health Care, as well as the development of new working methods. In this way pre-school Child Health Care will have a function at population level, a function that its workers, in close cooperation with others, will have to fill in. It seems justified to conclude that a (re)orientation of pre-school Child Health Care to environmental determinants demands a rather drastic innovation process. The recommendations given below have been formulated with this in view.

11.4 Recommendations

- For Child Health Care Policy:

    — The realization of a child health policy based on health objectives instead of health care objectives. In this way the influencing of environmental determinants will have direct relevance to the process of providing care.

    — The structural incorporation of population-level preventive tasks in pre-school Child Health Care.

- For the staff:

    — An adaptation of the range of duties of district nurses, so that besides work directed at individuals or groups, identification and active influencing of environmental determinants will be possible.

    — An adaptation of the range of duties of clinical medical officers, so that during the individual preventive visits explicit attention can be given to the recognition of health threatening environmental determinants and health profiles can be developed at community level (village, town). In this way, it will be possible for doctors to shoulder greater population-focused responsibility.

- For the organization:

— The creation of conditions within the organization which will allow the above mentioned policy to be established. This may include the creation of personal, financial and legal scope for such duties, the development of forms of cooperation, as well as the development of the required expertise among the staff.

— The development of a registration system that allows the recognition and inventory of health threatening environmental factors. Cooperation with the Municipal Health Services would seem evident here.

References

Bosma, M.W.M. & Hosman, C.M.H.: *Preventie op waarde geschat*, Nijmegen 1990.

Brinkgreve, C. & Regt, A. de: Het verdwijnen van de vanzelfsprekendheid. Over de gevolgen van individualisering voor kinderen, *Jeugd en Samenleving* 20 (1990) 5, 324–333.

Bronfenbrenner, U.: Ecology of the Family as a Context for Human Development: Research Perspectives, *Developmental Psychology*, 22 (1986) 723–742.

DeMause, L.: *The History of Childhood*, London: Souvenir Press, 1976.

Dungen, M. van den: Het Broeikaseffect. Gezin en samenleving rond 2000, *Gezin* 1 (1989) 3, 164–180.

Geelen, H., Kessels, J., Vorstermans, M.: *Netwerken voor jeugdhulpverlening. Een methodiek voor preventieve jeugdhulpverlening op buurtniveau*, Amersfoort: Acco, 1989.

GG&GD Amsterdam: *Vergelijkend buurtonderzoek naar sterfte, ziekenhuisopname en langdurige arbeidsongeschiktheid in Amsterdam*, Amsterdam: Instituut voor Sociale Geneeskunde, 1980.

GG&GD Amsterdam: *Maatwerk en werkmaat. Deelnota 1: zuigelingenen kleuterzorg*, Amsterdam 1990.

Hermanns, J.M.A.: *Het sociale kapitaal van jonge kinderen*, Utrecht: SWP, 1992 (oratie).

Liljeström, R.: The Public Child, the Commercial Child and our Child, in:

Kessel, F. & Siegel, A.W. (eds.): *The Child and other Cultural Inventions*, New York: Praeger, 1983.

Ministerie van WVC: *Opvoedingssteun op maat. Hoofdlijnen pedagogische preventie in het kader van het jeugdbeleid*, Den Haag: Sdu Uitgeverij, 1992.

Norbeck, H.J., Nijhuis, H.G.J., Egmond, J. van: Perinatale zuigelingensterfte in 's Gravenhage, *Epidemiologisch Bulletin's Gravenhage* 18 (1983) 1, 2–13.

Nijhuis, H.G.J.: Maatschappelijke omgeving, gezondheid en jeugdgezond-heidszorg, in: Bos, M.W. & Winter, M. de (red.): *Jeugdgezondheidszorg in de toekomst*, Lisse: Swets en Zeitlinger, 1989, pp.23–34.

Projectgroep Geïntegreerd Jeugdbeleid Almere/Projectgroep Gezonde Flevo-steden: *Atlas over de Jeugd in Almere*, Almere/Lelystad 1992.

Rutter, M.: Early Sources of Security and Competence, in: Bruner, J.H. & Garton, A. (eds.): *Human Growth and Development*, Oxford: Clarendon Press, 1978.

Rutter, M.: The City and the Child, *American Journal of Orthopsychiatry* 51 (1981) 610–625.

Wilbrink-Griffioen, D. & Eyck, A.M. van: *Preventie van opvoedingsproblemen*, Leiden: Research voor Beleid, 1990.

Winter, M. de: *Het Voorspelbare Kind. Vroegtijdige onderkenning van ontwikkelingsstoornissen (VTO) in wetenschappelijk en sociaal-historisch perspectief*, Lisse: Swets & Zeitlinger, 1986 (dissertation).

Winter, M. de: *De Kwaliteit van het Kinderlijk bestaan*, Bunnik 1990 (oratie).

WRR (Wetenschappelijke Raad voor het Regeringsbeleid): *De ongelijke verde-ling van gezondheid: verslag van een conferentie*, Den Haag 1987.

Index